Our Heritage

A Compact History of
Cardiac
Surgery

Our Heritage

A Compact History of
Cardiac
Surgery

A Sampath Kumar

MBBS, MS, MCh (Cardiothoracic Surgery)

Ex-Professor and Head
Department of Cardiothoracic
and Vascular Surgery
and Chief, Cardiothoracic Sciences Center
All India Institute of Medical Sciences
New Delhi, India

W Gerald Rainer

MD, MS (Surgery)

Distinguished Clinical Professor of Surgery
University of Colorado Health Sciences Center
Denver, Colorado, USA

CBS Publishers & Distributors Pvt Ltd

New Delhi • Bengaluru • Chennai • Kochi • Kolkata • Mumbai
Hyderabad • Nagpur • Patna • Pune • Vijayawada

Disclaimer

Science and technology are constantly changing fields. New research and experience broaden the scope of information and knowledge. The authors have tried their best in giving information available to them while preparing the material for this book. Although, all efforts have been made to ensure optimum accuracy of the material, yet it is quite possible some errors might have been left uncorrected. The publisher, the printer and the authors will not be held responsible for any inadvertent errors, omissions or inaccuracies.

Our Heritage

A Compact History of
Cardiac Surgery

ISBN: 978-81-23928-60-9

Copyright © Authors and Publisher

First Edition: 2017

Published by Satish Kumar Jain and produced by Varun Jain for

CBS Publishers & Distributors Pvt Ltd

4819/XI Prahlad Street, 24 Ansari Road, Daryaganj, New Delhi 110 002, India.
Ph: 23289259, 23266861, 23266867   Website: www.cbspd.com
Fax: 011-23243014   e-mail: delhi@cbspd.com; cbspubs@airtelmail.in.
Corporate Office: 204 FIE, Industrial Area, Patparganj, Delhi 110 092
Ph: 4934 4934   Fax: 4934 4935   e-mail: publishing@cbspd.com;
                                        publicity@cbspd.com

Branches

- **Bengaluru:** Seema House 2975, 17th Cross, K.R. Road, Banasankari 2nd Stage, Bengaluru 560 070, Karnataka
  Ph: +91-80-26771678/79   Fax: +91-80-26771680   e-mail: bangalore@cbspd.com
- **Chennai:** 7, Subbaraya Street, Shenoy Nagar, Chennai 600 030, Tamil Nadu
  Ph: +91-44-26680620, 26681266   Fax: +91-44-42032115   e-mail: chennai@cbspd.com
- **Kochi:** Ashana House, No. 39/1904, AM Thomas Road, Valanjambalam, Ernakulam 682 018, Kochi, Kerala
  Ph: +91-484-4059061-65   Fax: +91-484-4059065   e-mail: kochi@cbspd.com
- **Kolkata:** 6/B, Ground Floor, Rameswar Shaw Road, Kolkata-700 014, West Bengal
  Ph: +91-33-22891126, 22891127, 22891128   e-mail: kolkata@cbspd.com
- **Mumbai:** 83-C, Dr E Moses Road, Worli, Mumbai-400018, Maharashtra
  Ph: +91-22-24902340/41   Fax: +91-22-24902342   e-mail: mumbai@cbspd.com

Representatives

- **Hyderabad** 0-9885175004 • **Nagpur**   0-9021734563 • **Patna** 0-9334159340
- **Pune**   0-9623451994 • **Vijayawada** 0-9000660880

Printed at Rashtriya Printers, Dilshad Garden, Delhi, India

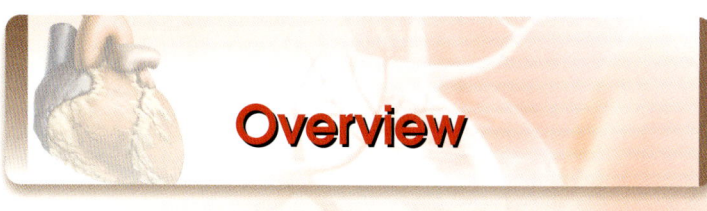

Overview

This is a ready reference book on history of cardiac surgery.

As a teacher and mentor to nearly a hundred super-speciality students, I have realized that trainees are not inclined to read history. They have large textbooks (in 3 volumes) and are hard pressed for time. Books on history of cardiac surgery currently in circulation offer detailed description of events, surgeons and their biographies. Trainees preparing for the certification examination need a quick reference book that provides answers to most questions on history in their examinations.

A book of this nature is a ready-reckoner for the practical examination. It can refresh teachers for their didactic lectures, presentations, etc. The format is simple with a photograph and a brief one-page description of contributions, locations, etc. This is perhaps the only way to interest the students and trainees to learn history of cardiac surgery.

It has taken nearly two years to find, download, obtain permissions to reproduce, write the brief citation, etc. of more than 100 physicians and surgeons for this book.

A Sampath Kumar

Foreword

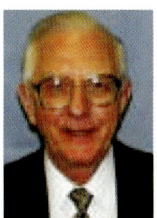

Dr Sampath Kumar has compiled certain pertinent biographical data on 109 individuals that he has chosen to include in this group of outstanding contributors to the field of cardiac surgery. Instead of formatting this book into a lengthy, detailed (and sometimes boring) account of the "ultimate biography" of these pioneers, he has purposely chosen a formula of photographs, abbreviated notes to place the person in context and with references for the reader to explore further if he/she so wishes. For the busy student, practitioner, or any interested reader, this is a quick reference designed to pique the interest of those concerned with the historical evolution of our speciality. Choosing personalities to enter into such a book as this involves a certain degree of personal prejudice and this is the prerogative of the author. Dr Kumar has certainly used his own personal tastes and preferences in this selection process and the result shows a wide representation of interests—some intimately involved with surgery itself and others who have played peripheral, albeit important roles, in the development of our speciality. This book deserves a special place on the reference-shelf of those individuals who have a feeling for history and its impact on what and why we do things as we do today. Kudos to Dr Kumar for helping to keep the spark of historical curiosity alive.

W Gerald Rainer

Preface

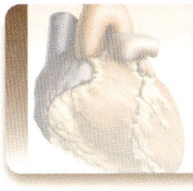

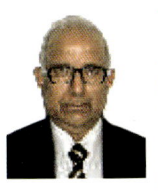

In four decades as teachers, we have found that students rarely study the history. History is the basis of our current practice. The developments in all aspects of cardiac surgery have come about because of an inherent need to find a suitable technique, a remedy, an innovation to provide relief to the patient suffering from heart disease. The bold and fearless attempts by pioneers provide a fascinating insight into the evolution of cardiac surgery. To we, this subject is the most interesting one to read.

Books on history recount the attempts of pioneers in great detail. The students, however, find a little time to read these detailed accounts during their training, particularly if the department is extremely busy performing a large number of procedures. As a consequence history of cardiac surgery takes a back seat in the curriculum and many teachers are equally unaware of these historic milestones.

This book attempts to fill this void. It is essentially a ready-reckoner for the student who seeks to identify these milestones with the pioneers. The book provides a photograph, a brief biography, location, contributions and one seminal reference. The interested student may then seek other select books on history to learn more details. It will be useful for the teacher as well as the student for immediate reference.

A Sampath Kumar • W Gerald Rainer

Contents

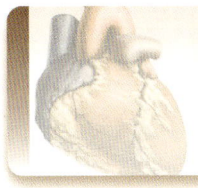

Our Heritage

A Compact History of
Cardiac
Surgery

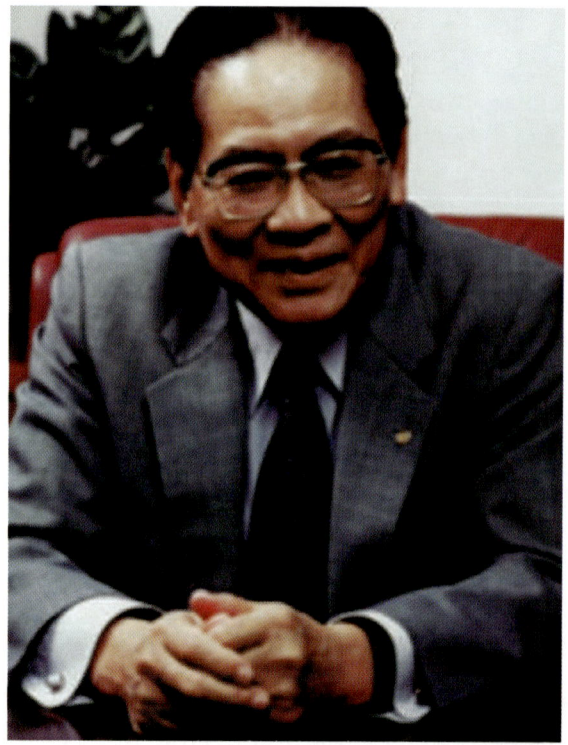

Theodore Akutsu

Reproduced with Permission from International J of Art Organs

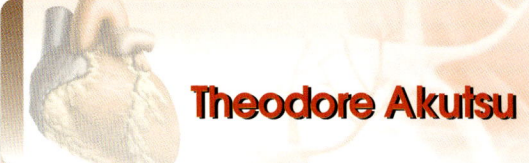

Theodore Akutsu

Dates : 20th August, 1922–9th August, 2007
Location : Cleveland Clinic, Cleveland, Ohio, USA

Contribution

- The first total artificial heart, developed along with Dr Kolff, implanted in a dog in 1957.

Interesting Fact

- 50 years later a heart replacement device was approved by FDA

Reference

Akutsu T and Kolff WJ, Permanent substitutes for valves and hearts, Trans Amer Soc Art Int Orgs 1958; 4: 230–232.

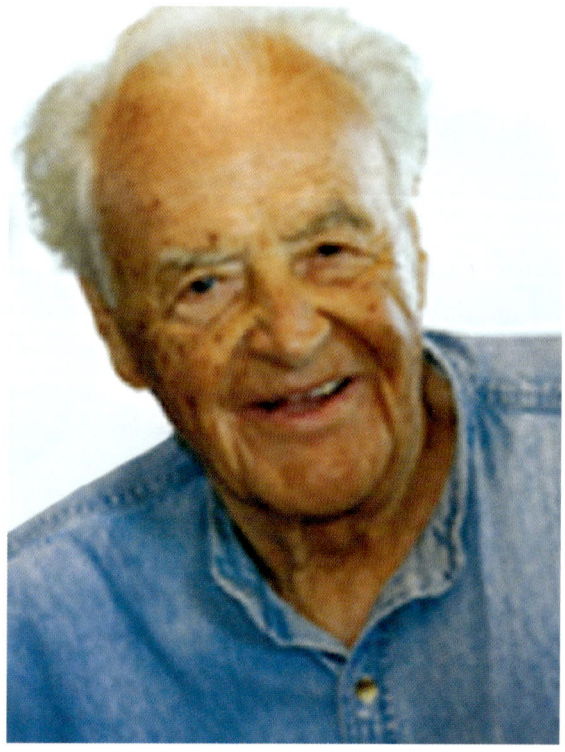

Kurt Amplatz

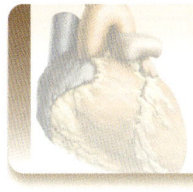

Kurt Amplatz

Born : 1924

Location : University of Minnesota, Minneapolis, Minnesota, USA

Contributions

- The Amplatz catheter for coronary angiography
- Dye injector for angiography
- Amplatzer occlusion device for transcatheter occlusion of atrial septal defects

Interesting Facts

- Was ordered to leave his workshop by a court of law
- Avid tennis player

Reference

Amplatz K, Ernst R, Lester RG, Lillehei CW, Lillie A., Retrograde left cardioangiography as a test of valvular competence, Radiology, Feb. 1959; 72(2): 268–9.

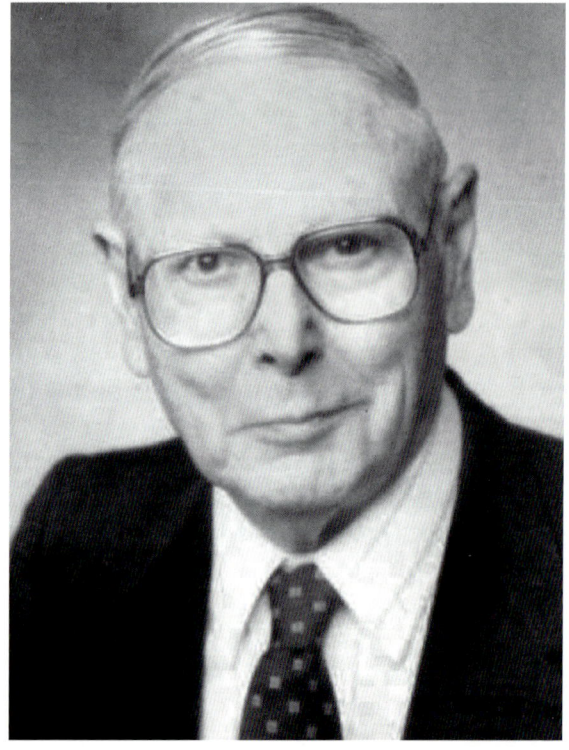

Charles Philamore Bailey

Courtesy of Gerald Rainer

Charles Philamore Bailey

Dates : 1911–18th August, 1993

Location : Hahnemann University Hospital, Philadelphia Pennsylvania, USA

Deborah Heart and Lung Institute, Browns Mills, New Jersey, USA

Contributions
- The first successful closed mitral valvotomy
- The beginning of direct heart surgery

Interesting Facts
- His rough, aggressive and volatile nature earned him a great deal of criticism
- Studied law and became a legal consultant

Reference
Bailey CP, Surgical treatment of mitral stenosis (mitral commissurotomy), Dis Chest, 1949; 15: 377–379.

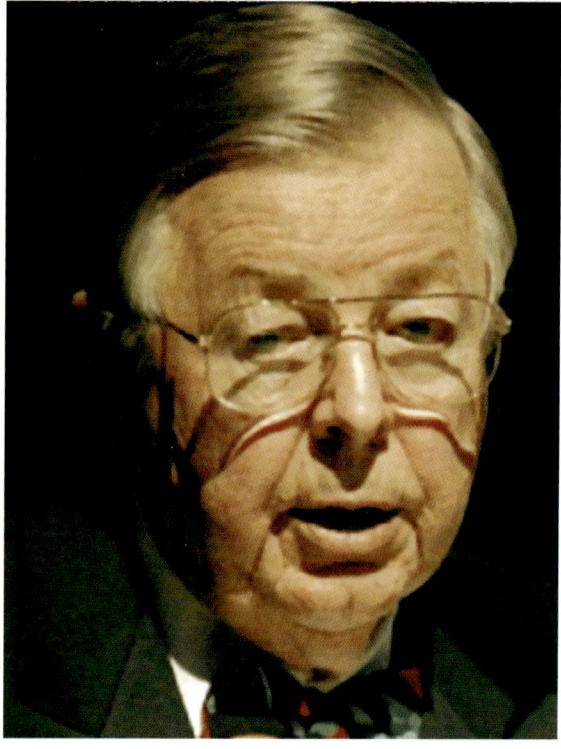

Earl E Bakken

Reproduced with Permission from Annals of Thoracic Surgery

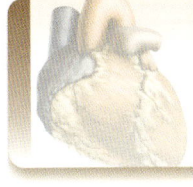

Earl E Bakken

Born : 10th January, 1924
Location : Minneapolis, Minnesota, USA

Contributions

- Invented and produced the first wearable external pacemaker for Dr C. Walton Lillehei in 1953
- Founded the Medtronic Corporation and produced with other doctors the first implantable pacemaker

Interesting Facts

- Driven to Bankruptcy he envisioned the Medtronic mission which is now the philanthropic division of Medtronic Inc.
- As a high school student developed a Taser to ward off bullies

Reference

Lillehei WC, Gott VL, Hodges PC, Long DM, Bakken EE, Transistor pacemaker for treatment of complete atrioventricular dissociation. JAMA, 1960; 172: 2006–2010.

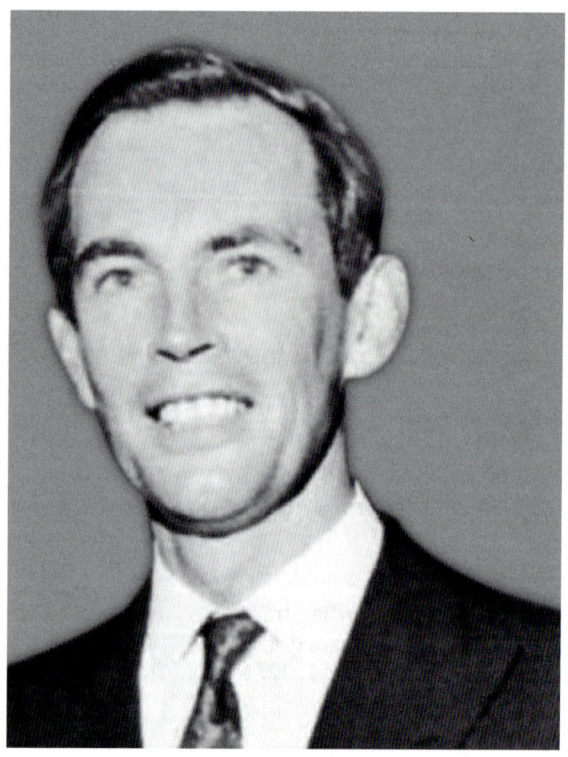

Christian Neethling Barnard

Courtesy of Gerald Rainer

Christian Neethling Barnard

Dates : 8th November, 1922–2nd September, 2001

Location : University of Capetown, South Africa

Contributions

- The world's first successful human heart transplantation December 3, 1967
- Performed several heterotopic heart transplants

Interesting Facts

- Has written several books
- Was known as "Film Star" surgeon

Reference

Barnard CN, A human cardiac transplant: An interim report of a successful operation performed at Groote Schuur Hospital, Cape Town, South Afr. Med J. 1967; 41:1271–1274.

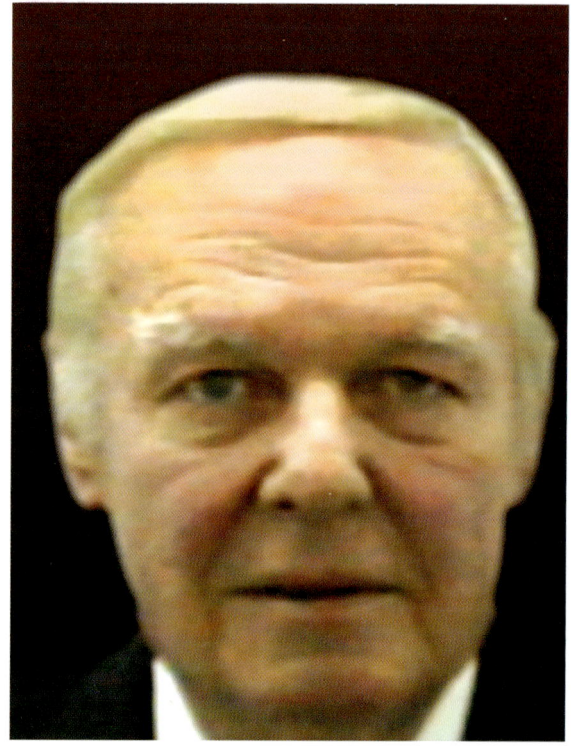

Arthur C Beall

Reproduced with Permission from CTS Net

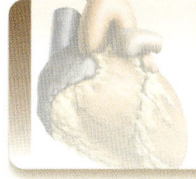

Arthur C Beall

Died   : 8th December, 2002

Location   : Baylor College of Medicine, Houston, Texas, USA

Contributions

- The Beall mechanical heart valve
- The introduction of arterial filters in the extracorporeal circuit

Interesting Fact

- His invention did not prove durable.

Reference

Beall AC Jr, George MC Jr, Cooley DA and DeBakey ME, J. Homotransplantation of the aortic valve, J. Thorac and Cardiovasc Surg. 1961; 42: 497–506.

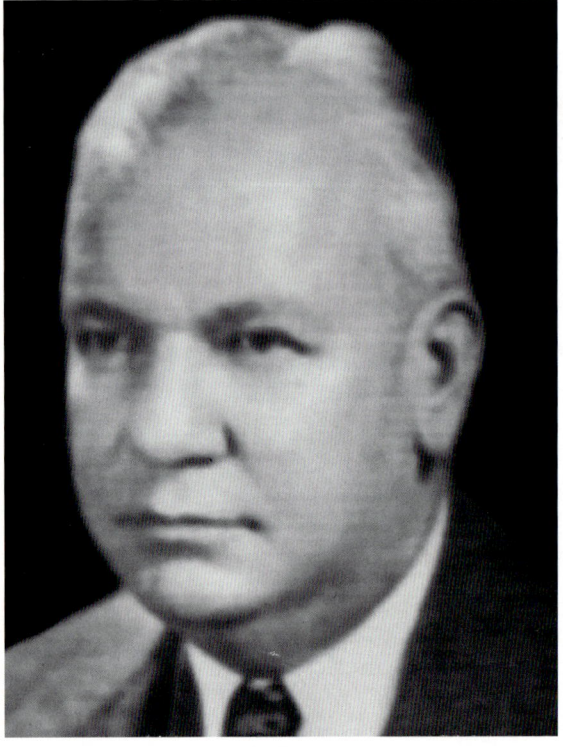

Claude Sehaeffer Beck

Courtesy of Gerald Rainer

Claude Sehaeffer Beck

Dates   : 1894–1971
Location   : University Hospitals of Cleveland,
                   Ohio, USA

Contributions

- Introduced operations to improve myocardial blood supply. The Beck I was to produce adhesions between pericardium and epicardium using talcum powder in 1935, Beck II where a saphenous vein graft was anastomised from aorta to coronary sinus 1940.
- First to use an internal defibrillator during a surgery on a 14-year-old boy in 1947.
- The "Beck's Triad" for recognition of cardiac tamponade.

Interesting Fact

- He was the first American Professor of cardiovascular surgery in 1952.

Reference

Beck CS, Resuscitation for cardiac standstill and ventricular fibrillation occurring during operation, Am J Surg, 1941; 54: 273–279.

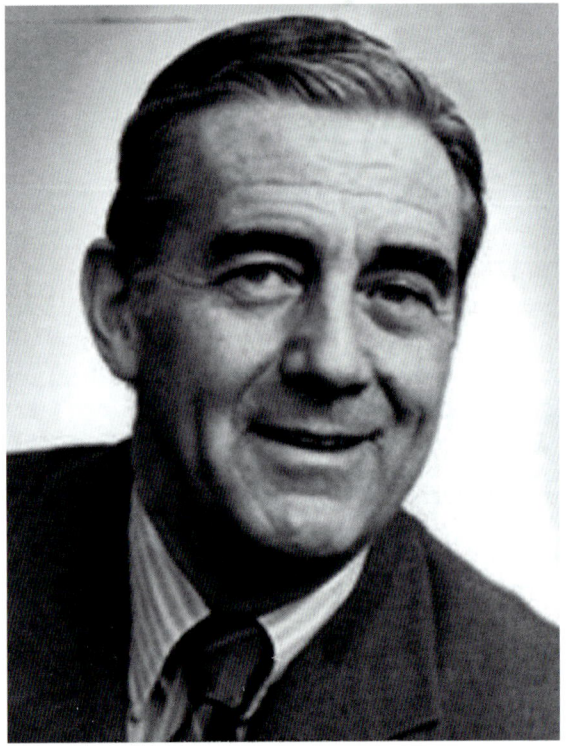

Wilfred Gordon Bigelow

Courtesy of Gerald Rainer

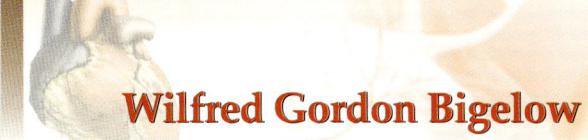

Wilfred Gordon Bigelow

Dates : 18th January, 1913–27th May, 2005
Location : University of Toronto, Toronto, Canada

Contribution

- Monumental study on effects of hypothermia and its metabolic effects. Resuscitation from hypothermic arrest

Interesting Facts

- Was Professor at Johns Hopkins in Baltimore
- Studied hibernation physiology in polar bears

Reference

Bigelow WG, Dolan FG and Campbell FW, The effect of hypothermia upon the risk of surgery, Sizieme congree de la soc. Int de chir. Copenhagen 1955; 631–644.

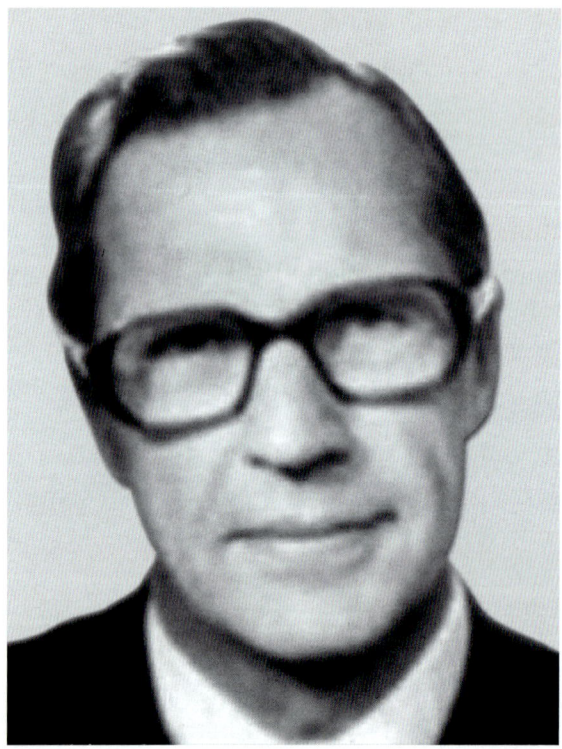

Viking Olov Bjork

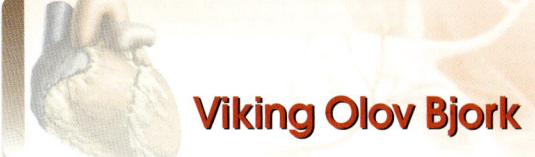

Viking Olov Bjork

Dates : 3rd December, 1918–8th February, 2009

Location : Karolinska Institute, Stockholm, Sweden

Contributions

- The Heart Lung Machine 1948 used in Experiments on animals
- The first left heart catheterisation in 1952
- The Bjork Shiley Heart Valve 1969

Interesting Fact

- His wife was his surgical assistant in his experiments on extracorporeal circulation in dogs.

Reference

Bjork VO, Aortic valve replacement with the Bjork-Shiley tilting disc valve prosthesis, Brit heart J. 1971; 33 (Suppl): 42–46.

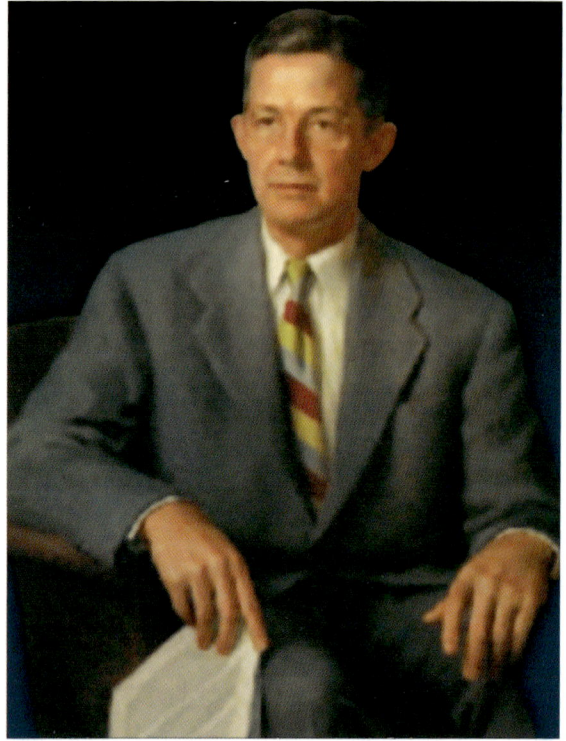

Alfred Blalock

Courtesy of Dr Duke Cameron, Johns Hopkins Hospital

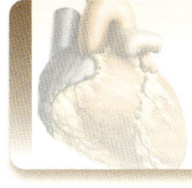

Alfred Blalock

Dates	:	5th April, 1899–15th September, 1964
Location	:	Johns Hopkins Hospital, Baltimore

Contributions

- The Blalock Taussig operation for blue babies in 1944.
- Trained a number of other pioneering surgeons.

Interesting Fact

- Played ping pong

Reference

Taussig HB, Blalock A, Observations on the volume of the pulmonary circulation and its importance in the production of cyanosis and polycythemia, Amer heart J, 1947; 33: 413–419.

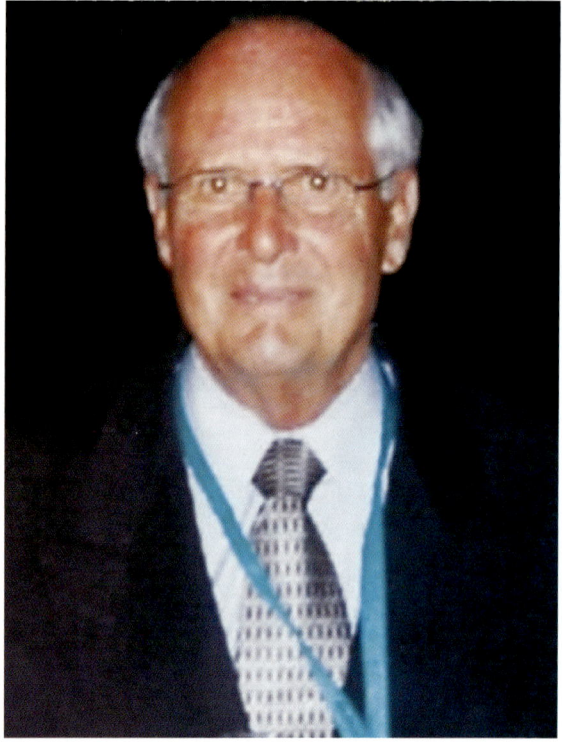

Sir Brian Barratt Boyes

A personal collection

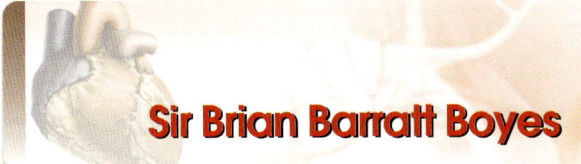

Sir Brian Barratt Boyes

Dates : 13th January, 1924–8th March, 2006

Location : Greenlane Hospital, Auckland, New Zealand Trained at Mayo Clinic and at University of Boston

Contributions

- Introduced the aortic homograft for AVR in 1962
- Produced enviable results in infants undergoing open heart surgery with profound hypothermia and circulatory arrest

Interesting Fact

- Decorated with CBE (Commander of British Empire) and KBE (Knight Commander of British Empire)

Reference

Barratt-Boyes BG, Simpson MM and Neutze JM, Intracardiac surgery in neonates and infants using deep hypothermia, Circulation 1971; 43: 125–130.

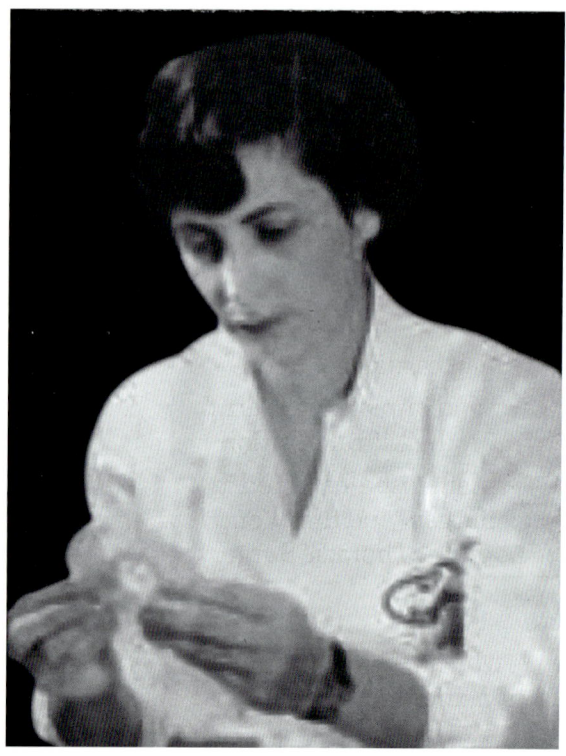

Nina Starr Braunwald

Reproduced with Permission from Annals of Thoracic Surgery

Nina Starr Braunwald

Dates   : 1928–1992

Location : George Town University, Mass, US

National Heart, Lung and Blood Institute (NHLBI), Bethesda, MD, USA

Contributions

- First woman cardiac surgeon
- Designed and implanted an artificial heart valve for the first time in the Mitral position in 1960
- First woman to be certified by American Board of Thoracic Surgery and first woman member of American Association for Thoracic Surgery.

Interesting Fact

- A gentle woman who successfully combined a demanding profession and bringing up a family.

Reference

Braunwald NS, Theodore C and Morrow AG, Complete replacement of the mitral valve. Successful clinical application of a flexile polyurethane prosthesis, J Thorac Cardiovasc Surg 1960; 41: 12–16.

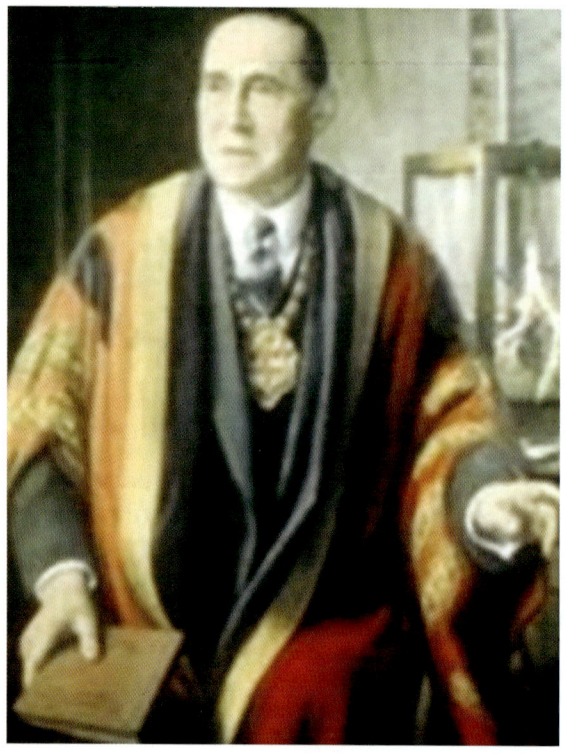

Lord Russell Claude Brock
(Lord Brock of Wimbledon)

Reproduced with Permission from Annals of Thoracic Surgery

Lord Russell Claude Brock
(Lord Brock of Wimbledon)

Dates   : 24th October, 1903–3rd September, 1980
Location : The Guy's Hospital, London, UK

Contributions
- The anatomy of the bronchial tree
- The treatment of congenital pulmonary stenosis

Interesting Fact
- He was a difficult task master to work with outside but was kind and generous inside.

Reference
Brock RC, Pulmonary valvulotomy for the relief of congenital pulmonary stenosis, Brit Med J, 1948; 1: 1121–1126.

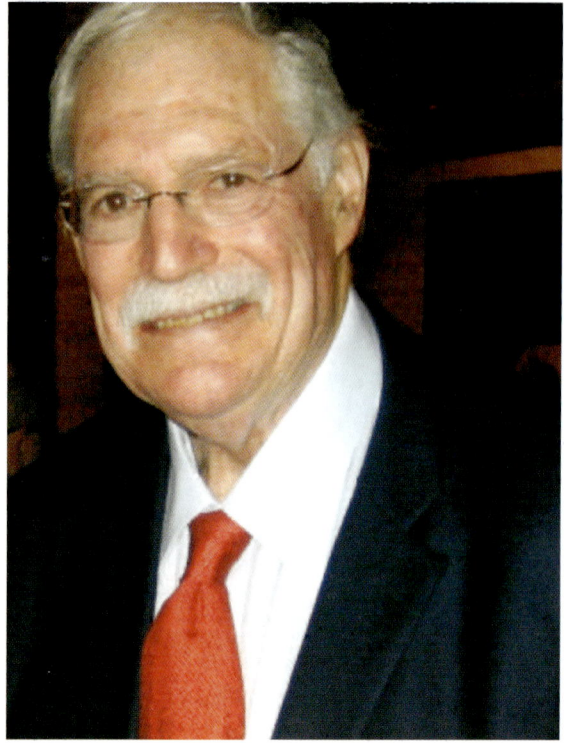

Gerald David Buckberg

Personal collection

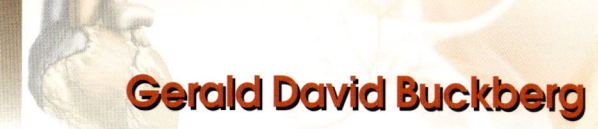

Gerald David Buckberg

Born   : 1935

Location : University of California at Los Angeles
(UCLA), Los Angeles, California, USA

Contributions

- Developed the principles and practice of Myocardial protection and the use of cardioplegia
- New concepts in the structure of the heart and the causes of heart failure

Interesting Fact

- Trained at Johns Hopkins Hospital

Reference

Follette DM, Mulder DG, Maloney JV, Buckberg GD. Advantages of blood cardioplegia over continuous coronary perfusion or intermittent ischemia: Experimental and clinical study, J. Thor Cardiovasc Surg 1978; 78: 604–619.

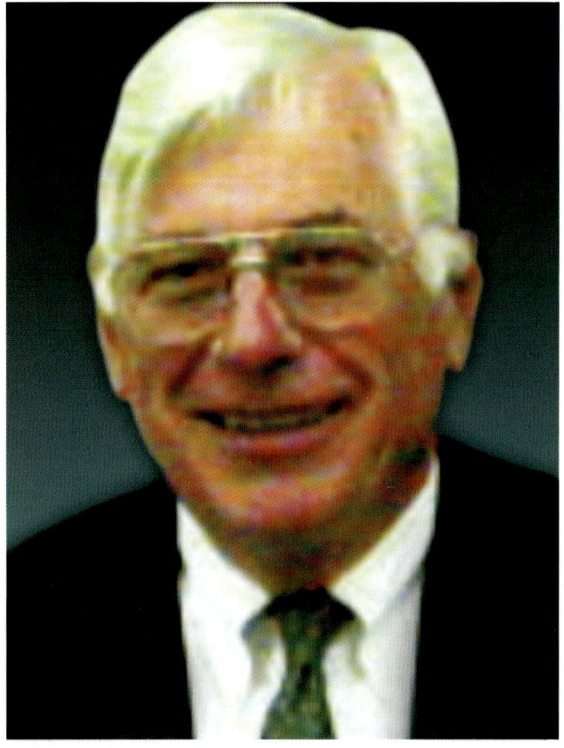

Mortimer J Buckley

Reproduced with permission from CTSNet

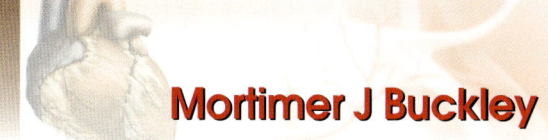

Mortimer J Buckley

Died   :   24th November, 2007

Location   :   Massachusettes General Hospital, Boston, Ma, USA

Contributions

- The clinical application of intra-aortic balloon pump
- The aggressive management of cardiogenic shock and mechanical complications of myocardial infarction

Interesting Facts

- Helped develop cardiac surgical units/centers in China, Venezuela and Korea
- Although feared in the operating room, he was a wonderful human being

Reference

Buckley MJ and Austen WG, Theoretical and experimental analysis of the intra-aortic balloon pump, Trans Am Soc Artif Int Orgs 1963; 14: 338–343.

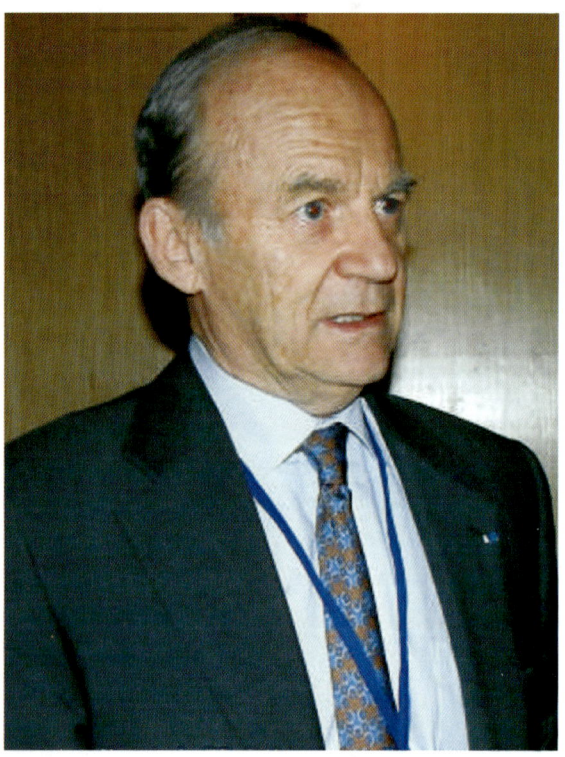

Alain Frederic Carpentier

Personal collection

Alain Frederic Carpentier

Born : 11th August, 1933

Location : Hopital Broussais, Paris, France, Hospital European Georges Prompidou, Paris

Contributions

- The principle technique of mitral valve repair
- The introduction of retrograde cardioplegia
- The operation for cardiomyoplasty
- The use of radial artery in CABG
- Design and fabrication of tissue heart valves

Interesting Fact

- Is now working on producing an artificial heart

References

Carpentier A, Branchini B, Cour JC, Asfaou E, Vallani M, Deloche A, Relland J, d Allaines CI, Blondeau Ph, Pawnica A, Parenzan L and Brom G. Congenital malformations of the mitral valve in children. Pathology and surgical treatment, J Thorac Cardiovasc Surg 1976; 72: 854–866.

Carpentier A, Lemaigre G, Robert L, Carpentier S, Dubost C, Biological factors affecting long term results of valvular heterograft, J. Thor Cardiovasc Surg 1969; 58: 467–483.

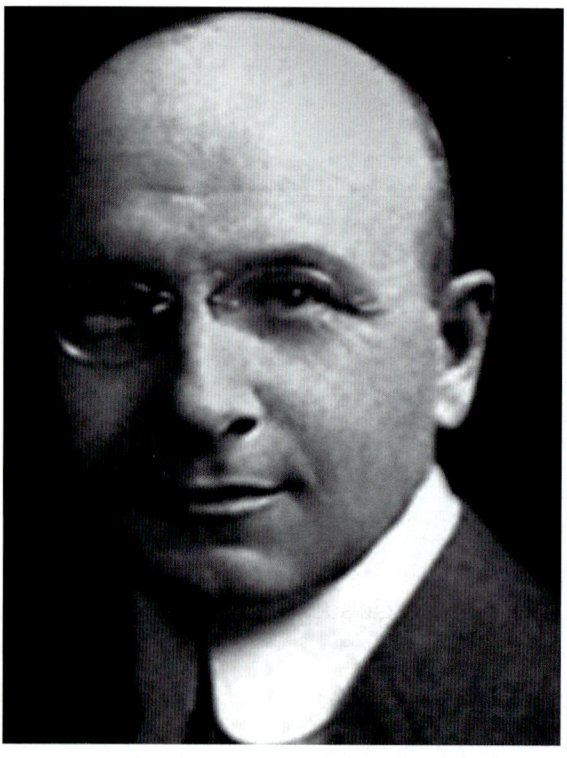

Alexis Carrel

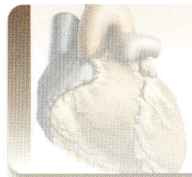

Alexis Carrel

Dates : 28th June, 1873–5th November, 1944

Location : University of Lyons, Lyons General Hospital, Lyons, France
Rockfeller Institute, New York, USA

Contributions

- Experimental research on transplantation of organs and tissues
- End to end anastomosis of arteries in 1902
- Successful valvotomies on the heart with Theodore Tuffier

Interesting Fact

- Only cardiothoracic surgeon to receive Nobel Prize in Medicine in 1912

Reference

Carrel A, Experimental surgery of the thoracic aorta and the heart, Ann Surg 1910; 52: 83–95.

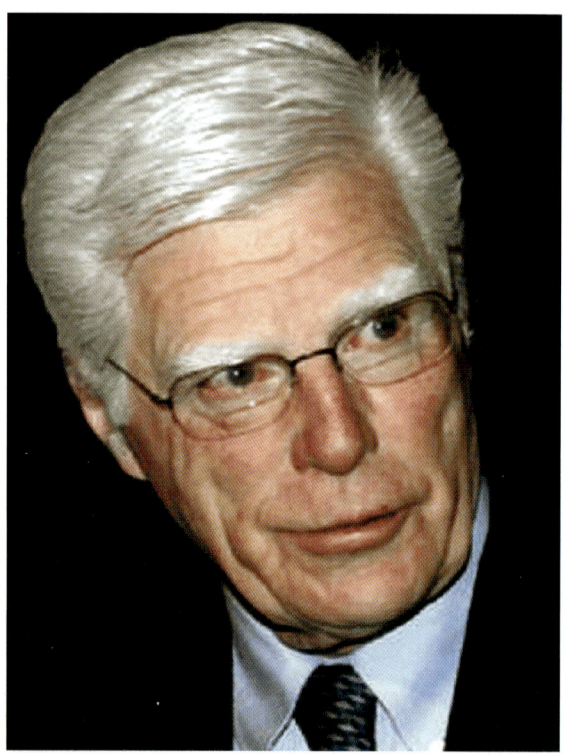

Aldo R Casteneda

Reproduced with permission from Annals of Thoracic Surgery

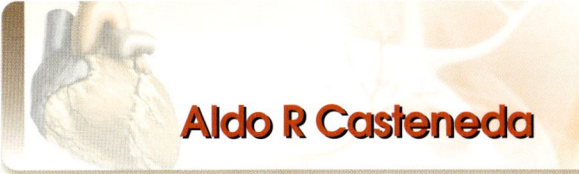

Aldo R Casteneda

Born : 1930

Location : University of Minnesota, Boston
Children's Hospital, Boston, Massachusetts,
USA, Guatemala City, Guatemala.

Contributions

- The introduction of deep hypothermia and circulatory arrest for repair of complex congenital heart lesions
- The concept of early correction in the neonate of all congenital anomalies

Interesting Fact

- He succeeded Robert Gross as Chief of Cardiovascular Surgery.

Reference

Castaneda AR, Arn A, Habelmann SP, Muller JH, Zamora R, Cardiopulmonary autotransplantation in primates, J Cardiovasc Surg 1972; 13: 523–531.

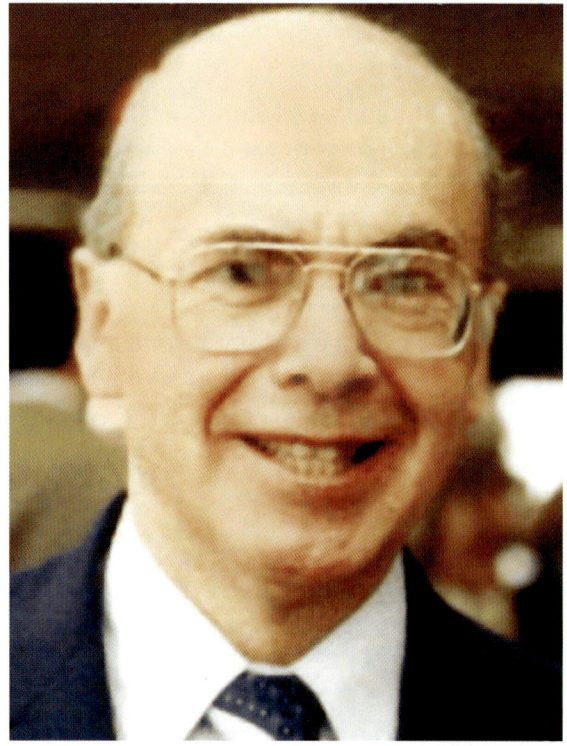

Morley Cohen

Reproduced with permission from Annals of Thoracic Surgery

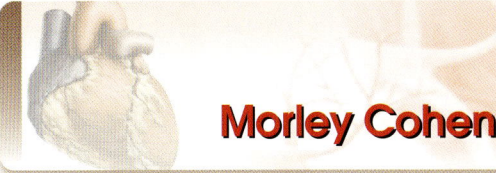

Morley Cohen

Dates	:	18th November, 1925–18th August, 2005
Location	:	Boniface General Hospital, University of Manitoba

Contribution

- With Walton C. Lillehei—for the first series of intracardiac surgeries with controlled cross circulation

Interesting Fact

- Was co-inventor of oxygenator.

Reference

Cohen M and Lillehei CW, Autogenous lung oxygenation with total cardiac bypass for intracardiac surgery, Surg Forum, 1954; 4: 34–40.

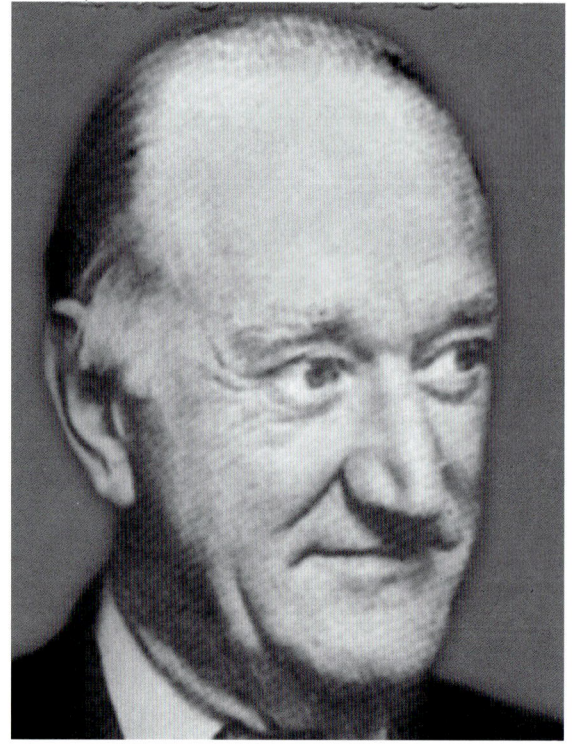

John Leigh Collis

Permission from IJTCVS

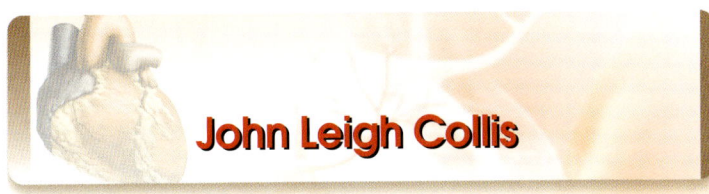

John Leigh Collis

Dates : 1911–4th February, 2003

Location : Birmingham General Hospital, UK
Brompton Hospital, UK

Contributions

- Esophageal resection in early 1930s with a low morbidity
- Mitral valvotomies and lung resections in India, at the Military Hospital in AUNDH, near Pune

Interesting Fact

- Used fine fuse wire as sutures

Reference

Collis JL, An Operation for Hiatus Hernia with Short Oesophagus, Thorax. September 1957; 12: 181–188.

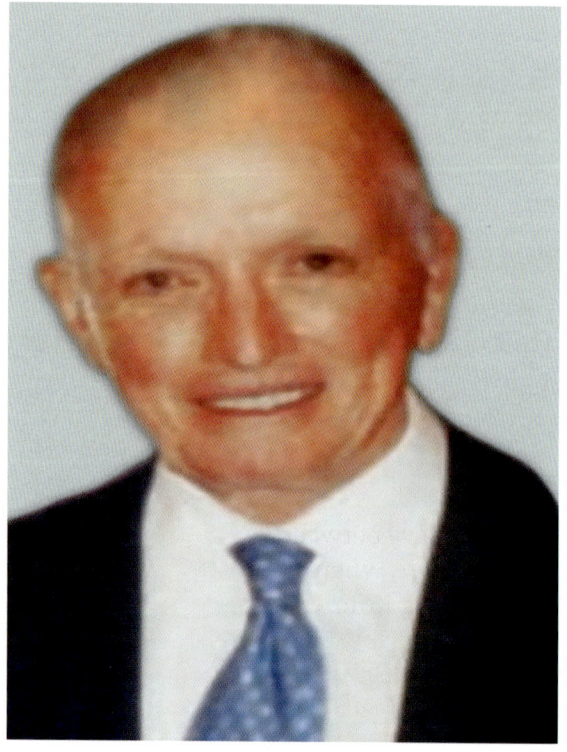

Denton Arthur Cooley

Personal collection

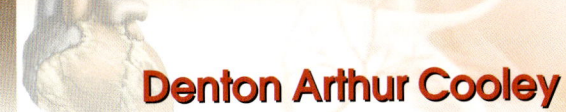

Denton Arthur Cooley

Born : 22nd August, 1920

Location : Texas Heart Institute, Houston, Texas, USA

Contributions

- Largest experience in heart surgery
- First successful heart transplant in USA in 1968
- First successful implantation of a total artificial heart in Man

Interesting Fact

- A 55-year-rivalry between Cooley and Dr DeBakey was resolved in 2007, when he presented DeBakey with the Texas Heart Institute Award.

Reference

Cooley DA, Bloodwell RD, Hallman GL, James NJ, Gunyon HM, Organ transplantation for advanced cardiopulmonary disease, Ann Thorac Surg 1969; 8: 36–40.

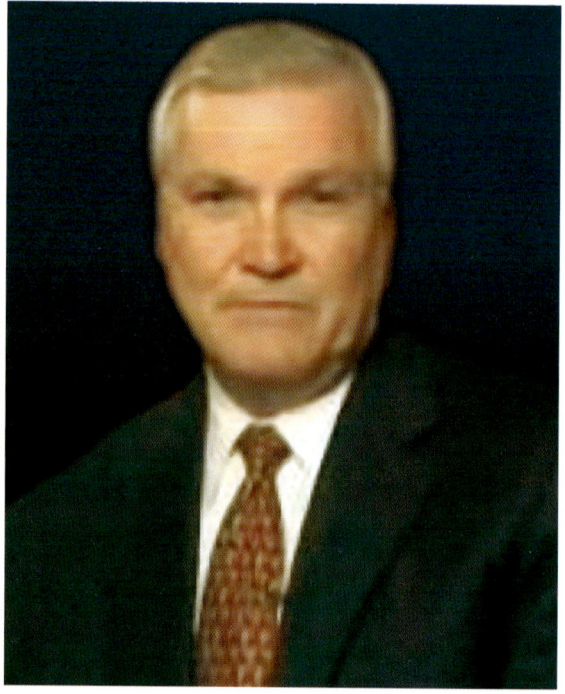

James L Cox

Personal collection

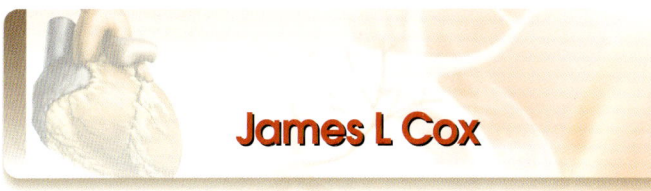

James L Cox

Born   : 24th December, 1942

Location : Washington University School of Medicine, St. Louis, Missouri

Contribution

- The identification, description and successful surgical conversion of atrial fibrillation to sinus rhythm—the Cox Maze Procedure.

Interesting Fact

- Now lives in a horse ranch with family

Reference

Cox JL, The surgical treatment of atrial fibrillation IV. Surgical technique, J Thorac Cardiovasc Surg 1991; 101: 584–592.

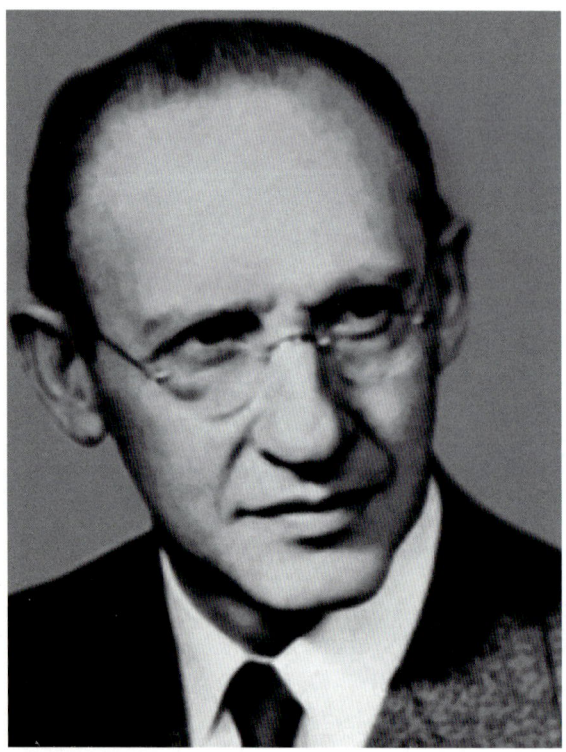

Clarence Crafoord

Courtesy of Gerald Rainer

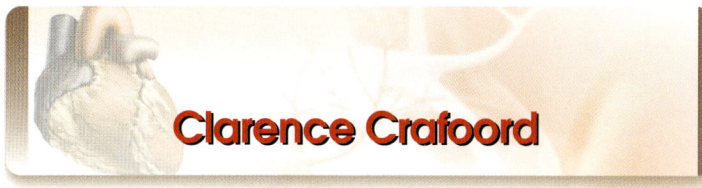

Clarence Crafoord

Dates : 1899–1984

Location : Karolinska Institute, Stockholm, Sweden

Contributions

- First successful repair of coarctation in a young boy, 19th October, 1944
- Developed a respirator
- Developed along with Bjork, a disc oxygenator

Interesting Fact

- Has done all surgeries except ophthalmic

Reference

Bjork G and Crafoord C, Arteriovenous aneurysm on the pulmonary artery simulating patent ductus arteriosus Botalli, Thorax, 1947; 2: 65–73.

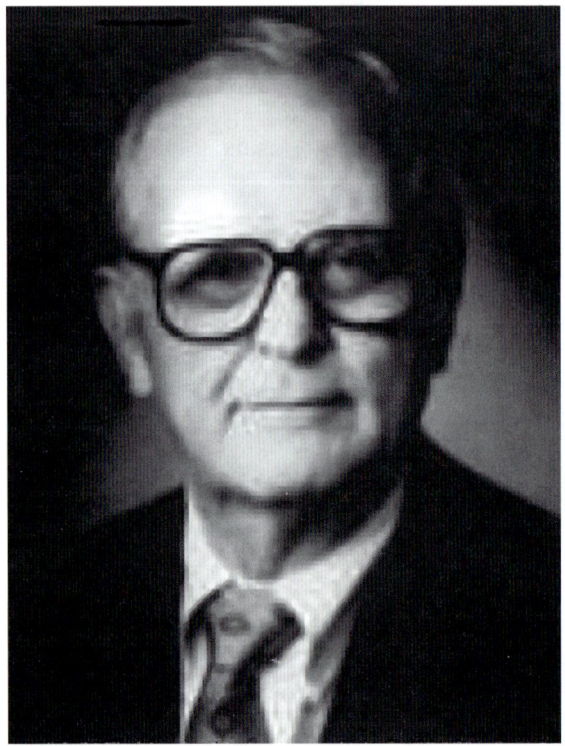

Earle Stanley Crawford

Reproduced with permission from Elsevier

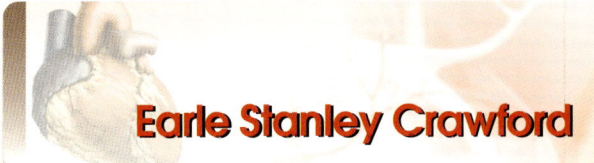

Earle Stanley Crawford

Dates : 1922–1992

Location : Baylor College and University of Houston, Texas, USA

Contributions

• The surgical treatment of aortic aneurysms—new and innovative techniques

• Transaortic mitral valve replacement

Interesting Fact

• Developed the cell saver for rapid retransfusion of shed blood

Reference

Crawford ES, Snyder DM, Cho GC, Roehm JOF, Progress in treatment of thoracoabdominal and abdominal aortic aneurysms involving celiac, superior mesenteric and renal arteries, Ann Surg, 1978; 188: 404–442.

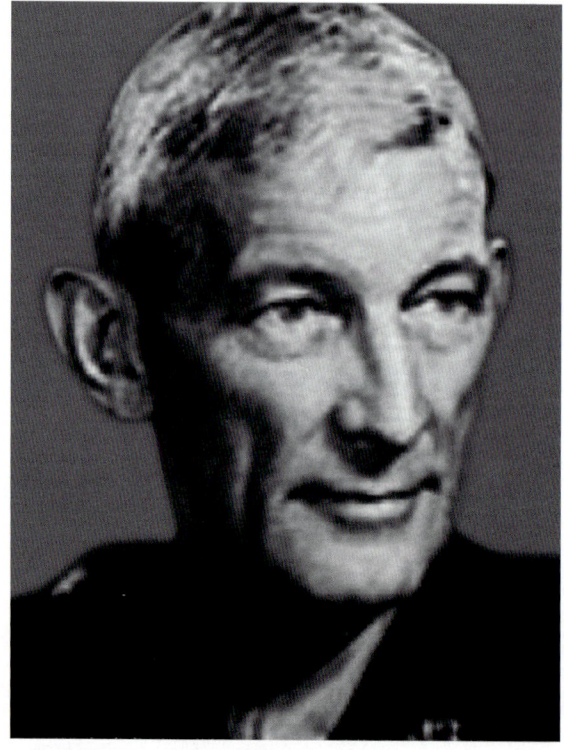

Elliot Carr Cutler

Courtesy of Dr Gerald Rainer

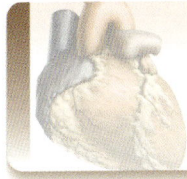

Elliot Carr Cutler

Dates : 30th July, 1888–16th August, 1947

Location : Harvard Medical School

Peter Bent Brigham Hospital Boston, Massachusetts, USA

Contributions

- Direct heart surgery for Mitral Stenosis in 1923, by finger fracture. This was later abandoned.
- He authored a textbook on *Atlas of Surgery with Zollinger* in 1939.
- Activist for humane treatment of experimental animals

Interesting Fact

- Was offered Professorship at Johns Hopkins by William Halstead but refused

Reference

A Cardiovalvulotome, Beck CS, Cutler EC, Laboratory of Surgical Research of Harvard Medical School, Boston, J Exp Med. 1924; 40: 375–379.

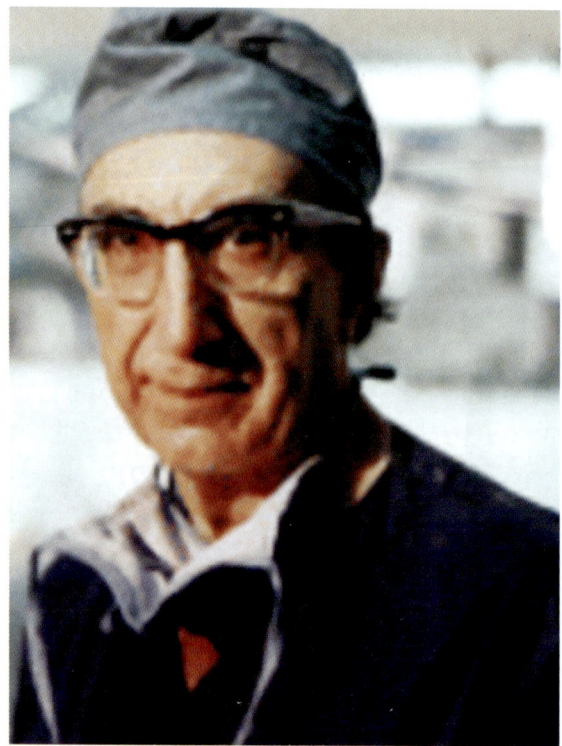

Michael Ellis DeBakey

Reproduced with permission from Annals of Thoracic Surgery

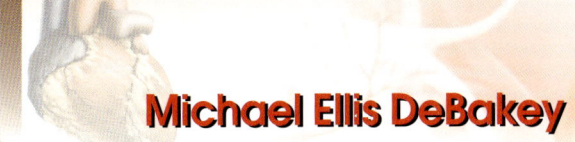

Michael Ellis DeBakey

Dates   : 7th September, 1908–11th July, 2008
Location : Baylor College of Medicine, Houston, Texas, USA

Contributions

- Invented the Roller pump at age 20
- Introduced vascular grafts—Dacron
- Invented surgical instruments for use of aorta—the "Atraumatic" grip is attributed to him
- Medical statesman— worked for developing the mobile army surgical hospital (MASH) and the veterans administration medical facilities
- Practiced medicine till his death (at just short of 100 years of age)
- Development and use of the first external heart pump
- First to record heart surgery on film

Interesting Facts

- Known as Texas Tornado, he was legendary for speeding
- Nearly lost his medical license in 1994
- Invited to supervise heart bypass on Russian President
- Underwent aortic surgery at the age of 97, the oldest patient to undergo such surgery recovered fully

Reference

De Bakey ME, Cooley DA, Successful resection of aneurysm of thoracic aorta and replacement by graft, JAMA 1953; 152; 673–676.

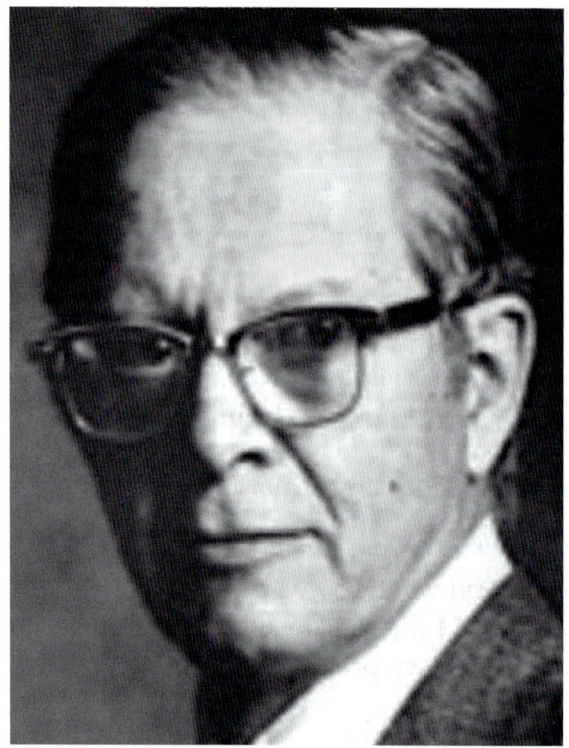

Clarence Dennis

Reproduced with permission from CTSNet

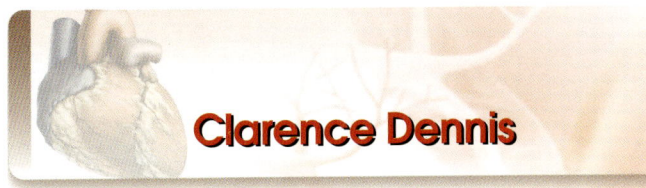

Clarence Dennis

Dates : 16th June, 1909–11th July, 2005

Location : University of Minneosota, Minneapolis, USA

State University of New York, Brooklyn, NY, USA

Contributions

- First heart lung machine in 1951
- Second successful ASD closure using the heart lung machine
- Dennis clamp for bowel anastomosis

Interesting Facts

- He invented whatever was needed to get the job done
- He invented a compact video camera for his own viewing, his own projection booth

Reference

Dennis C, Spreng DSJ, George NE, Karl KE, Russell NM, John TV, Phillip EW, Varco RL. Development of a pump oxygenator to replace the heart and lungs; an apparatus applicable to human patients, and applicable in one case, Ann Surg 1951; 134: 709–721.

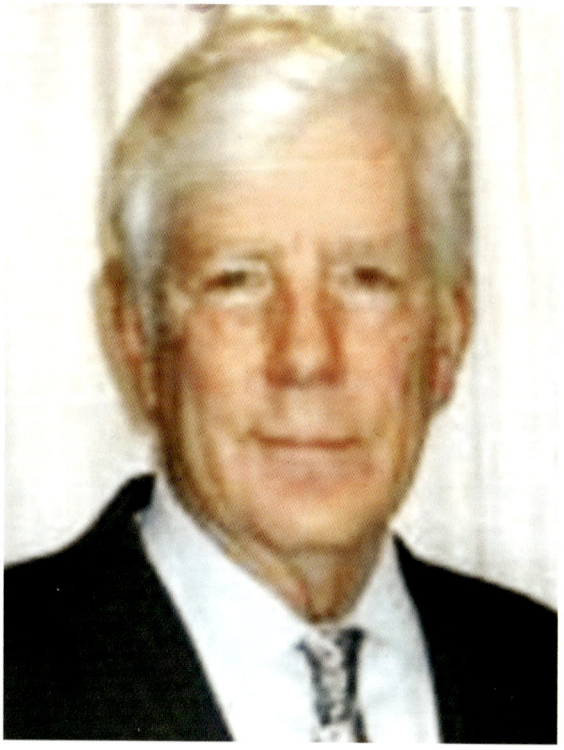

William C DeVries

Reproduced with permission from CTSNet

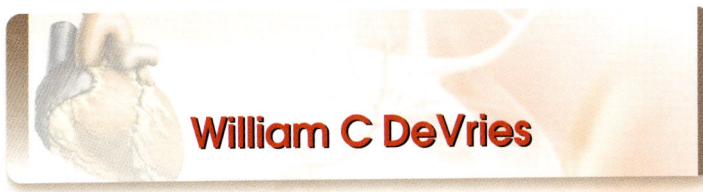

William C DeVries

Born : 19th November, 1943

Location : Walter Reed Memorial Hospital, Washington, USA

Contribution

- Implanted the first total artificial heart, the Jarvik 1 in 1984

Interesting Fact

- Joined the army as a Colonel at age 57 in 2000

Reference

De Vries WC, The permanent artificial heart. Four case reports, JAMA, 1988; 259: 849–859.

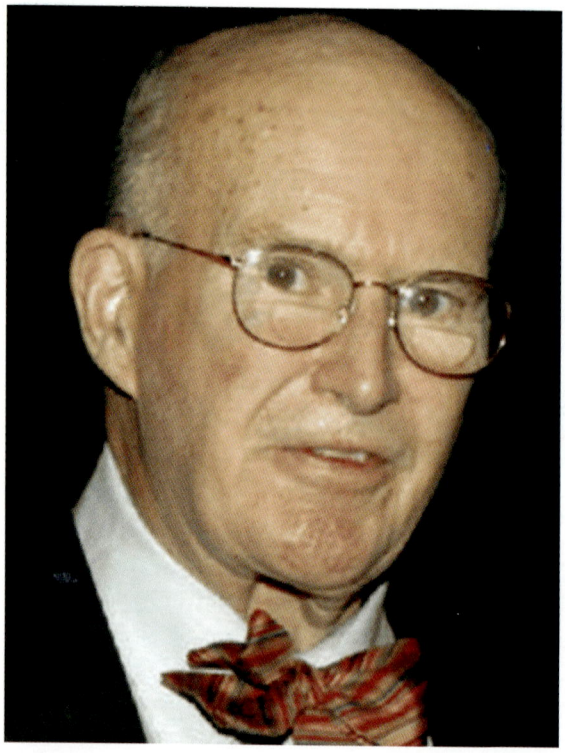

Richard A. DeWall

Reproduced with permission from Annals of Thoracic Surgery

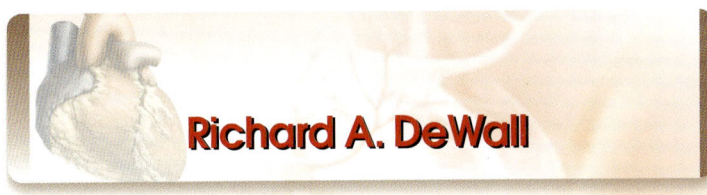

Richard A. DeWall

Dates : 16th December, 1926–15th August, 2016

Location : University of Minnesota, Minneapolis
Wright State University Medical School, Oakland, Ohio

Contribution

- Designed the first oxygenator which was used in an open heart surgery in 1955, along with Walton Lillehei.

Interesting Fact

- Produced the first workable oxygenator. Established School of Medicine in Wright State University.

Reference

De Wall RA, Warden HE, Read RC, et al., A simple expandable artificial oxygenator for open heart surgery, Surg Clin North Am, 1956; 36: 1025–1034.

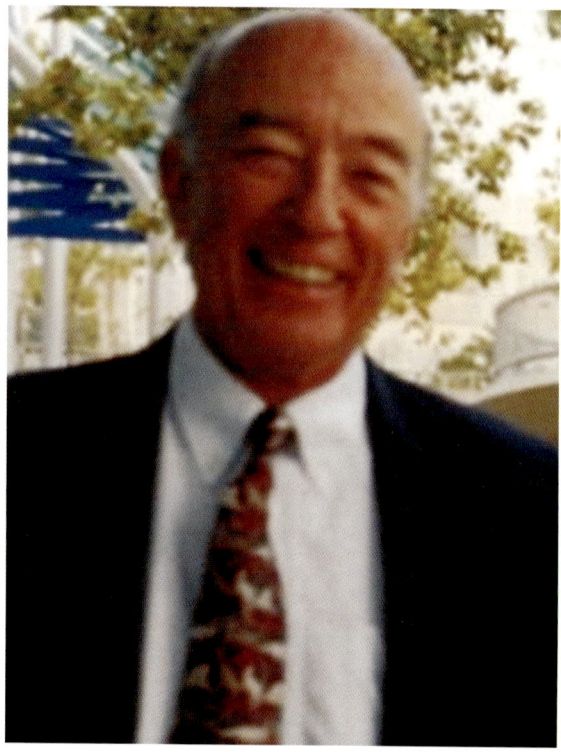

Carlos Gomez Duran

Personal collection

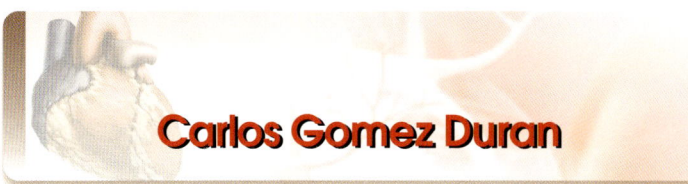

Carlos Gomez Duran

Born : June 1932

Location : University of Santander, Spain,
King Faisal Hospital, Saudi Arabia

International Heart Institute of Montana,
Missoula, Montana

Contributions

- Developed the use of aortic homograft
- Techniques in mitral valve repair
- Techniques in aortic valve repair

Interesting Facts

- Loves cruising
- Travelled coast to coast in US 3,000 miles by road

Reference

Duran CG, Gunning AJ, A method for placing a total homologous aortic valve in the subcoronary position, Lancet 1962; 2: 488–489.

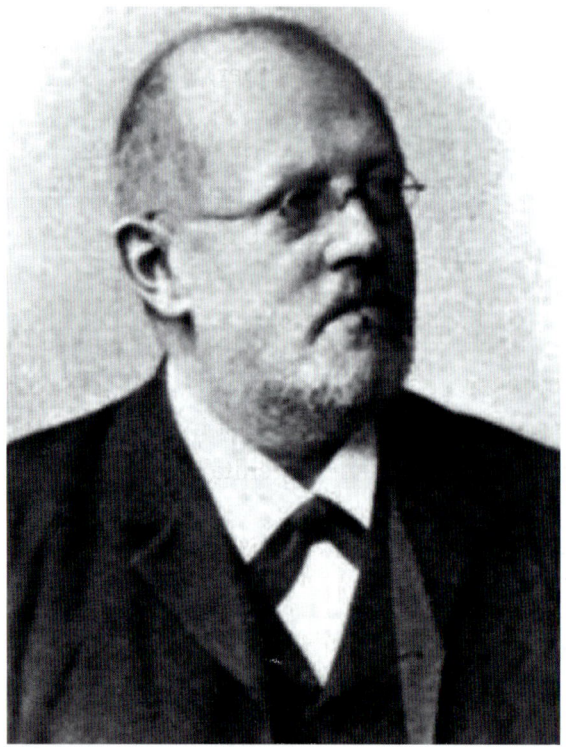

Wilhelm Ebstein

Internet/Wikipedia

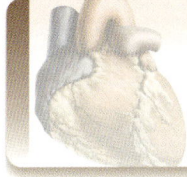

Wilhelm Ebstein

Dates : 27th November, 1836–22nd October, 1912

Location : University of Breslau and Berlin, Germany

Gottingen University, Gottingen, Germany

Contributions

- Considered a leading specialist in malnutrition
- In 1885 described the congenital cardiac anomaly that bears his name
- Also described a febrile illness known as Pel-Ebstein fever

Interesting Fact

- He recognised that fat contained two and half times as many calories as carbohydrates

Reference

Ebstein, W, Das Chronische Rückfallsfieber, eine neue infektionkrankheit Berlin Klin Wochensch, 1887; 24; 565–568.

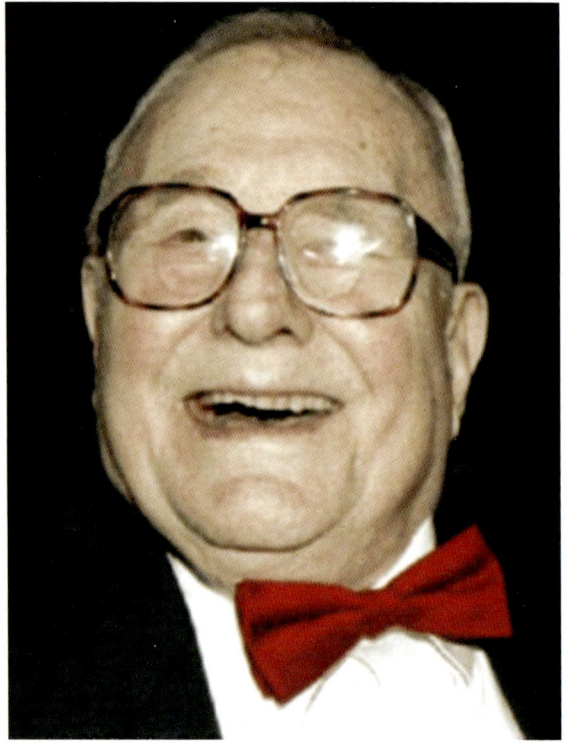

Jesse Efrem Edwards

Reproduced with permission from Annals of Thoracic Surgery

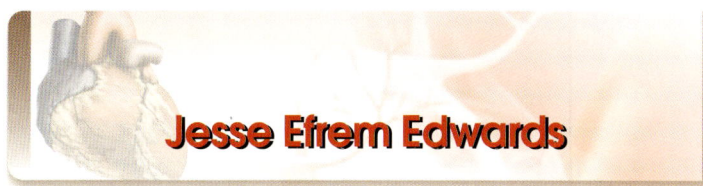

Jesse Efrem Edwards

Dates : 14th July, 1911–11th May, 2008

Location : Mayo clinic, Rochester, Minnesota, USA

University of Minnesota, St. Paul, MN USA

Contributions

- Description and classification of congenitally malformed hearts
- Had collected 2200 heart specimens, with two Atlases of congenitally malformed hearts
- Established the Edwards registry of cardiovascular diseases

Interesting Facts

- Testified against war crimes after World War II
- After a stroke learned to write with his left hand and wrote two books

Reference

Edwards JE and Buschell HB, Congenital tricuspid atresia: A classification, Surg Clin North Am 1949; 33: 1177–1196.

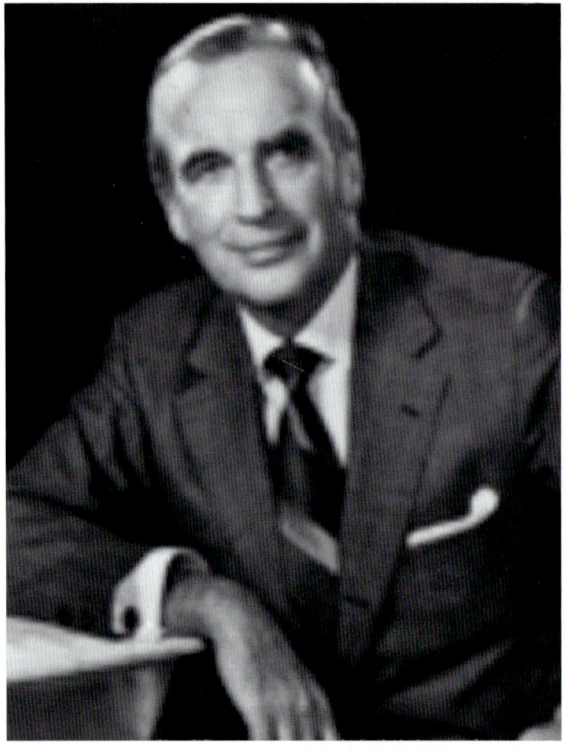

Donald B. Effler

Reproduced with permission from CTSNet

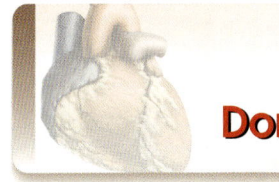

Donald B. Effler

Dates : 18th August, 1915–21st April, 2004

Location : Cleveland Clinic, Cleveland, OH USA

Contributions

- Direct coronary artery surgery using a patch graft in 1966.
- Open heart surgical correction of post infarction VSD using a heart lung machine developed by Willem Kolff.

Interesting Fact

- Helped establish the Philippine Heart Centre.

Reference

Kolff WJ, Effler DB and Groves LK, A review of four dreaded complications of open-heart operations, Br Med J. 1960; 16: 1149–1153.

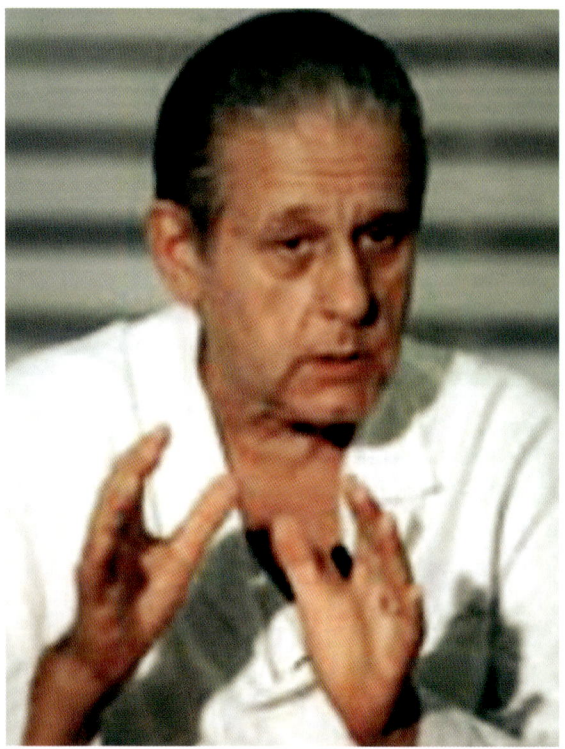

Rene Geronimo Favaloro

Courtesy of Gerald Rainer

Rene Geronimo Favaloro

Dates : 1923–2000

Location : Buenos Aires, Argentina, Cleveland Clinic, Cleveland, Ohio, USA

Contributions

- Was a rural physician for a number of years, reducing infant mortality and improving general health of community
- At the age of 40 he went to work as resident at Cleveland Clinic in USA and in May 1967 performed the first aorta coronary bypass in a 51-year-old lady
- Founded the Favaloro Foundation in Buenos Aires, Argentina for Medical Education and Research

Interesting Fact

- He committed suicide because of the enormous burden of loans

Reference

Favaloro RG, Saphenous vein autograft replacement of severe segmental coronary artery occlusion, Ann Thor Surg 1968; 5: 334–339.

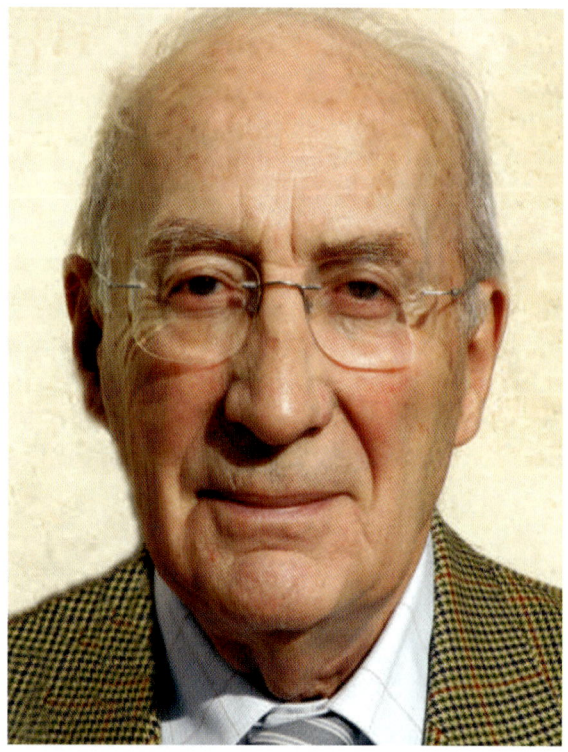

Francis Maurice Fontan

Personal collection

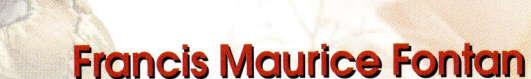

Francis Maurice Fontan

Born : 1929

Location : University of Bordeaux, Paris, France

Contribution

- Bypass of RV with Baudet 1971

Interesting Fact

- Produces wine

Reference

Fontan FM and Baudet E, Surgical repair of tricuspid atresia, Thorax, 1971; 26: 240–248.

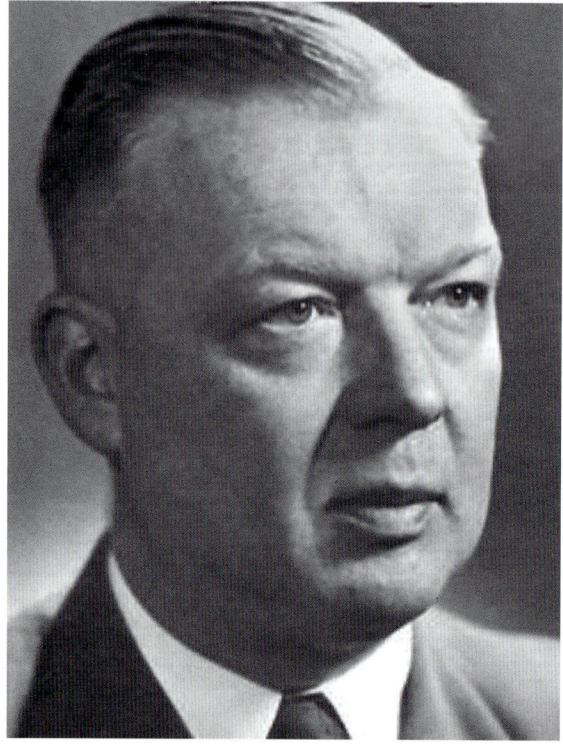

Werner Theodor Otto Forssmann

Courtesy of Gerald Rainer

Werner Theodor Otto Forssmann

Dates   : 29th August, 1904–1st June, 1979

Location : Evangelical Hospital, Dusseldorf, Germany

Honorary Professor of Surgery and Urology at Johannes Guterberg University, Mainz, Germany

Contribution

- Cardiac catheterisation which he performed on himself in 1929

Interesting Facts

- He was an urologist
- Nobel Prize in Medicine, 1956

Reference

Frossman WT, Catheterization of the right heart, Klinische Wochenschrift 1929; 8: 2085–2087.

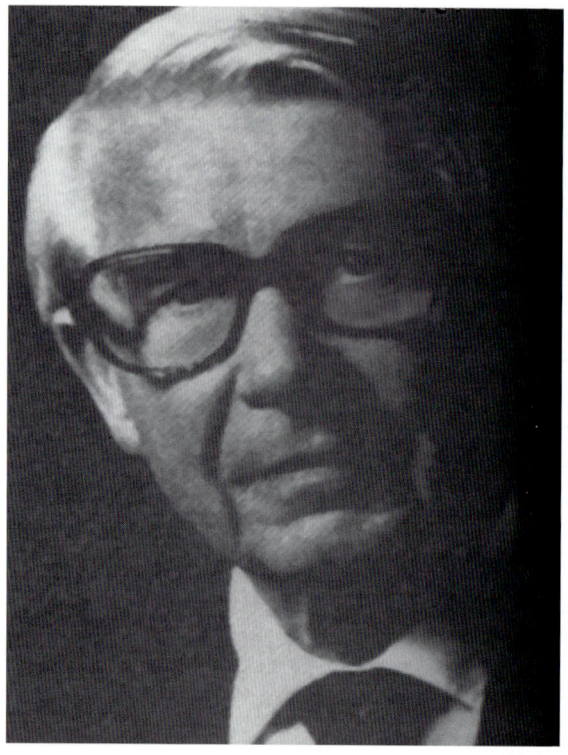

Frank Gerbode

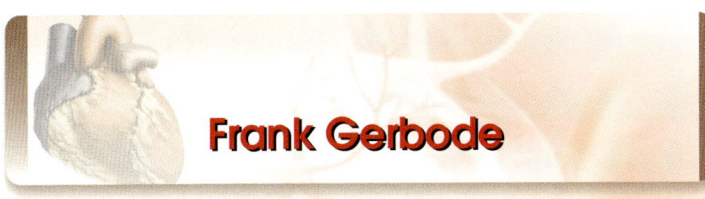

Frank Gerbode

Dates : 1907–1984

Location : California Pacific Medical Centre, San Francisco, California, USA

Contributions

- Described the left ventricle to right atrial shunt
- Established a research lab for developing the membrane oxygenator

Interesting Fact

- Trained nearly 200 fellows in his cardiovascular fellowship program

Reference

Gerbode F, The use of the enlarged left subclavian artery to overcome defects associated with complicated coarctation of the aorta, Surgery 1955; 37; 58–63.

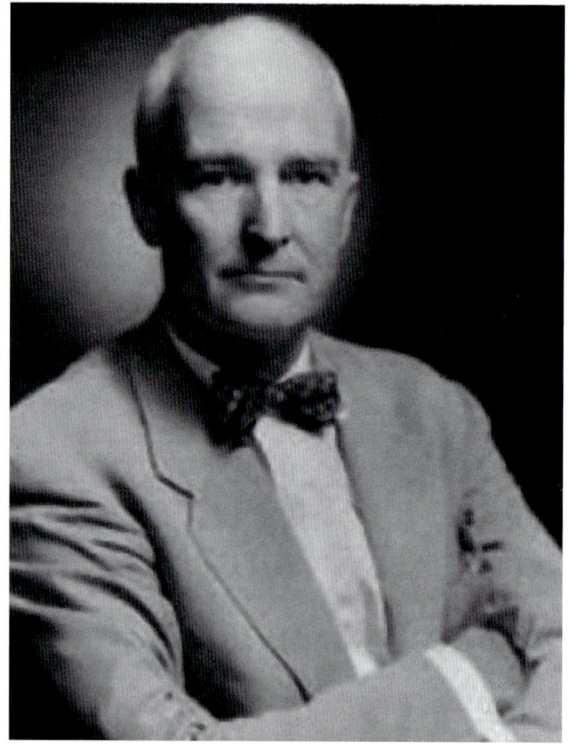

John H Gibbon Jr

Courtesy of Gerald Rainer

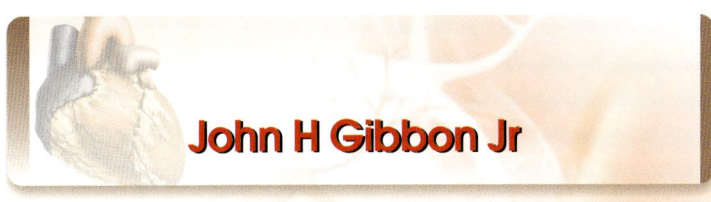

John H Gibbon Jr

Dates : 1903–1973

Location : Jefferson Medical College, Philadelphia, Pennsylvania, USA

Contributions

- Developed (invented) the heart lung machine
- Performed the first direct vision open heart surgery using the heart lung machine

Interesting Fact

- Dr Gibbon's machine failed to provide success in open heart surgery. He finally abandoned it.

Reference

Gibbon JH Jr, Artificial maintenance of circulation during experimental occlusion of pulmonary artery, Arch Surg 1937; 34: 1105–1131.

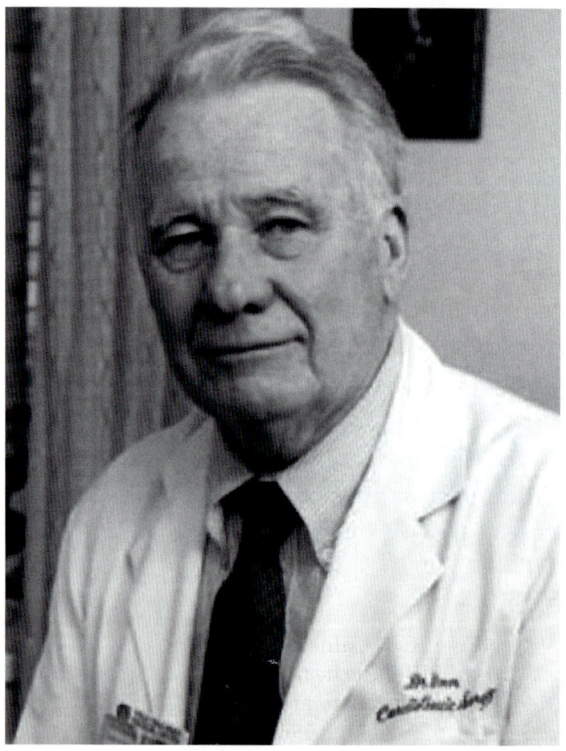

William Wallace Lumpkin Glenn

Reproduced with permission from Texas Heart Institute Journal

William Wallace Lumpkin Glenn

Dates   : 12th August, 1914–10th March, 2003

Location   : Yale University School of Medicine, Yale University

Contributions

- The Glenn shunt, superior vena cava to RPA—for blue babies
- Radiofrequency pacemaker and Diaphragm pacer

Interesting Facts

- Football fan
- Fond of fishing

Reference

Glenn WWL, Nelson OK, Talner NS and Edward CP, Circulatory bypass of the right side of the heart shunt between the superior vena cava and distal right pulmonary artery: Report of clinical application in thirty-eight cases, Circulation 1966; 31: 172–189.

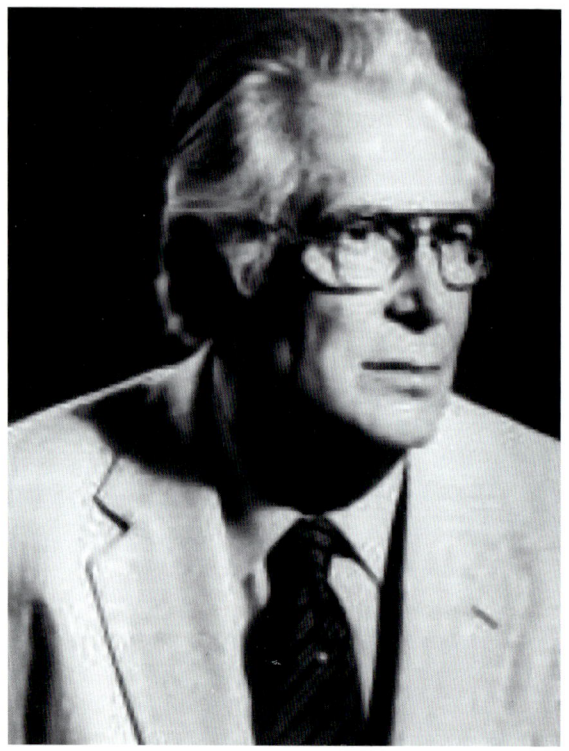

Robert Hans Goetz

Reproduced with permission from Annals of Thoracic Surgery

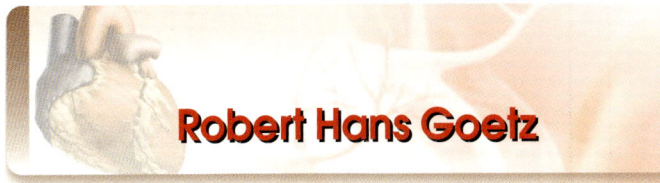

Robert Hans Goetz

Dates : 17th April, 1910–15th December, 2000

Location : Albert Einstein Medical Centre, Bronx, New York, USA

Contribution

- 1st successful coronary artery anastomosis, 2nd May, 1960—RIMA to RCA using a Tantalum ring

Interesting Facts

- Established a vascular research lab at Grute Schurr Hospital at Cape Town, South Africa
- Studied physiology of circulation in giraffes with a new technique of catheterisation

Reference

Haller JD, Kripke DC, Rosenak SS, Dee R, Roberts T, Rohman M and Goetz RH, Long term results of small vessel anastomoses with a ring. Ann Surg, 1965; 161: 67–72.

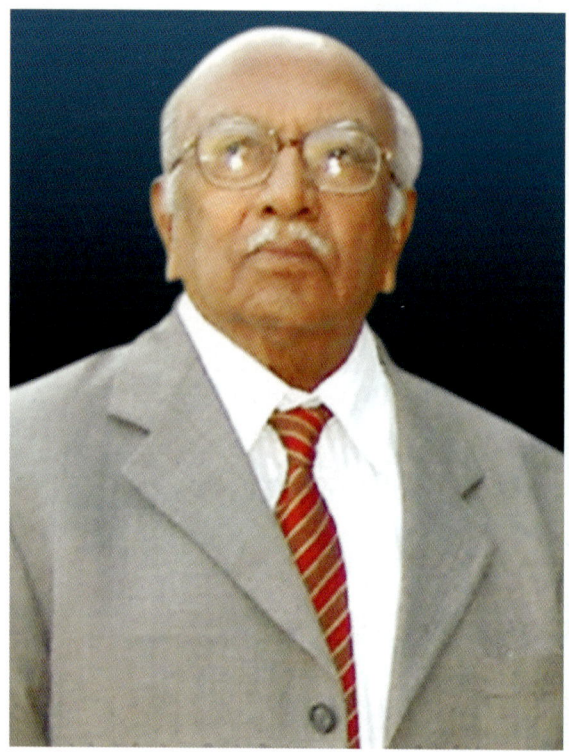

Nagarur Gopinath

Personal collection

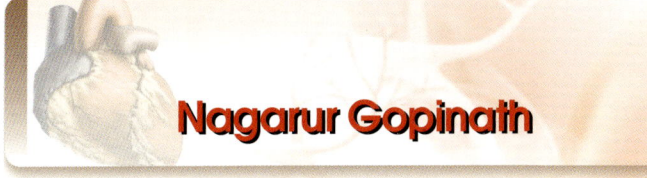

Nagarur Gopinath

Dates   :   November 1922–31st June, 2006
Location :   Christian Medical College, Vellore
                  All India Institute of Medical Sciences, Delhi

Contributions

- The first open heart surgery in India with hypothermia and later with cardiopulmonary bypass
- Established the heart centre at AIIMS
- Most experienced surgeon with pulmonary resection

Interesting Fact

- Along with Christian Barnard he trained with Walton Lillehei in Minneapolis

Reference

Cherian G, Vytilingam KI, Sukumar IP, and Gopinath N, Mitral valvotomy in young patients, Br Heart J. 1964: 26: 157–166.

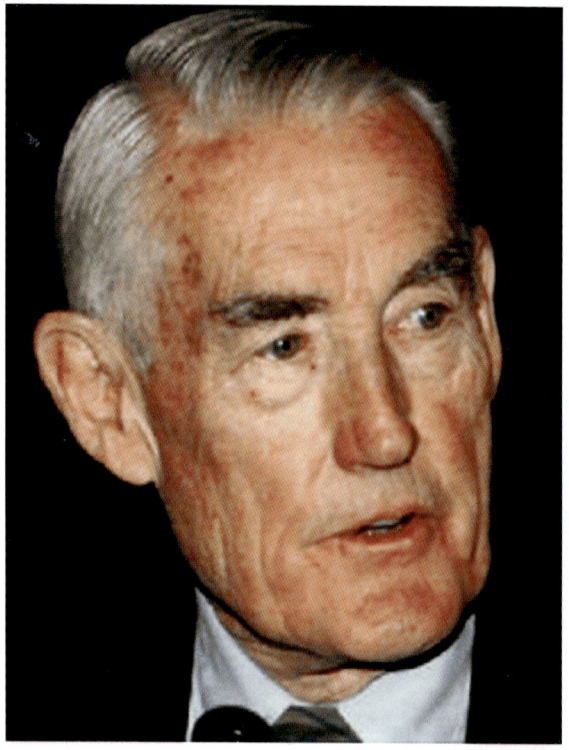

Vincent L. Gott

Reproduced with Permission from Annals of Thoracic Surgery

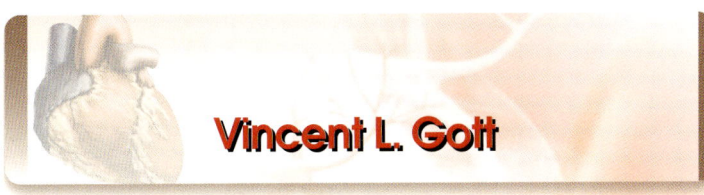

Vincent L. Gott

Born : 1927

Location : Johns Hopkins University, Baltimore, Maryland, USA

Division of Cardiac Surgery, the Institute of Genetic Medicine and the Howard Hughes Medical Institute, The Johns Hopkins Medical Institutions, Baltimore, Maryland 21287, USA

Contributions

- Gott shunt for aortic surgery.
- Designed the Gott-Daggett heart valve.
- Trained a number of cardiac surgeons.

Interesting Fact

- He was very good at illustrations of surgical operations and surgeons

Reference

Gott VL., et al. Replacement of the aortic root in patients with Marfan's syndrome, NEJM 1999; 340: 1307–1313.

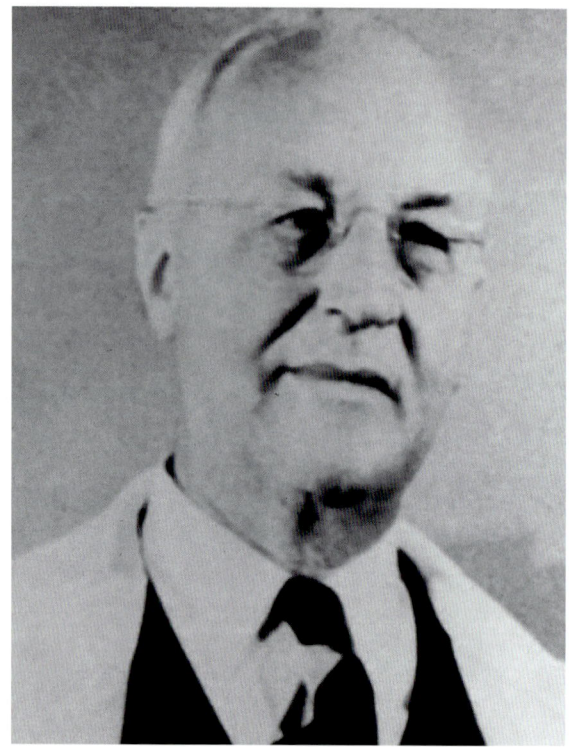

Evarts Ambrose Graham

Reproduced with permission from Interactive Journal Cardiovascular Surgery

Evarts Ambrose Graham

Dates : 19th March, 1883–4th March, 1957

Location : Washington University School of Medicine, St. Louis, USA

Contributions

- The relationship between smoking and lung cancer
- Pulmonary resection for lung cancer
- Helped establish The American Board of Surgery

Interesting Fact

- Died of lung cancer from smoking

Reference

Graham EA, Isaac B, Edward C and Leo E, War department, Guides in therapy for medical officers, US Technical manual 8–210, Washington DC, March 1942; 20: 185.

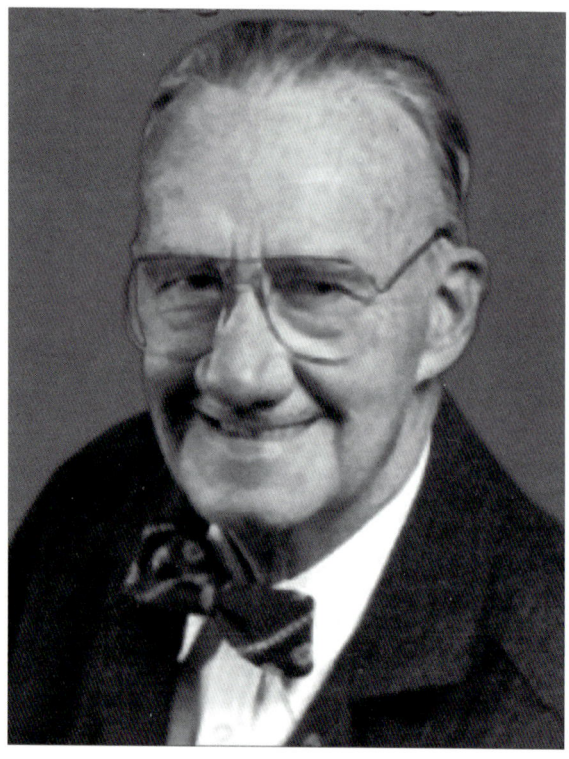

Wilson Greatbatch

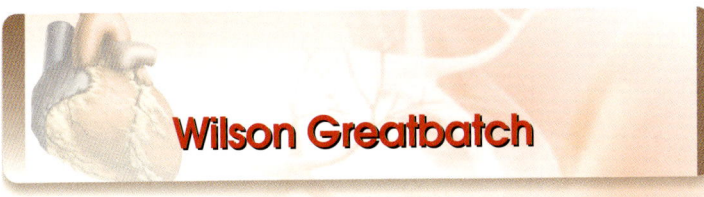

Wilson Greatbatch

Born : 1919

Location : Massachusetts Institute of Technology, Boston

Contributions

- Inventor of the implantable cardiac pacemaker—along with Dr Chardack

Interesting Fact

- US Airforce pilot who survived World War II

Reference

Chardack WM, Gage AA, Greatbatch W, A transistorized, self-contained, implantable pacemaker for the long-term correction of complete heart block, Surgery, Oct. 1960; 48: 643–654.

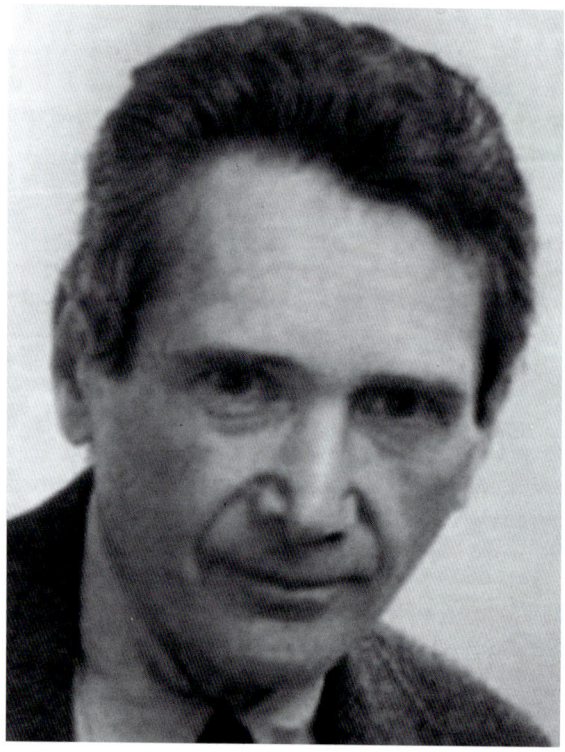

George Green

Personal collection

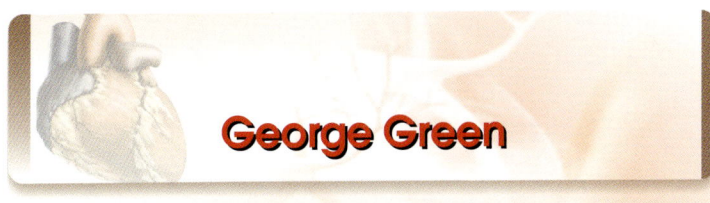

George Green

Born	:	18th January, 1932
Location	:	Professor of Surgery, Columbia University, New York Yale University trained

Contributions

• Performed the first LIMA-LAD bypass in February 1968 in humans

Interesting Fact

• Was a head and neck surgeon, used microsurgery techniques that led him to experiment with IMA-LAD anastomosis

Reference

Spencer FC, Green GE, Tice DA, and Glassman E, Bypass grafting for occlusive disease of the coronary arteries: a report of experience with 195 patients, Ann Surg. 1971; 173: 1029–1044.

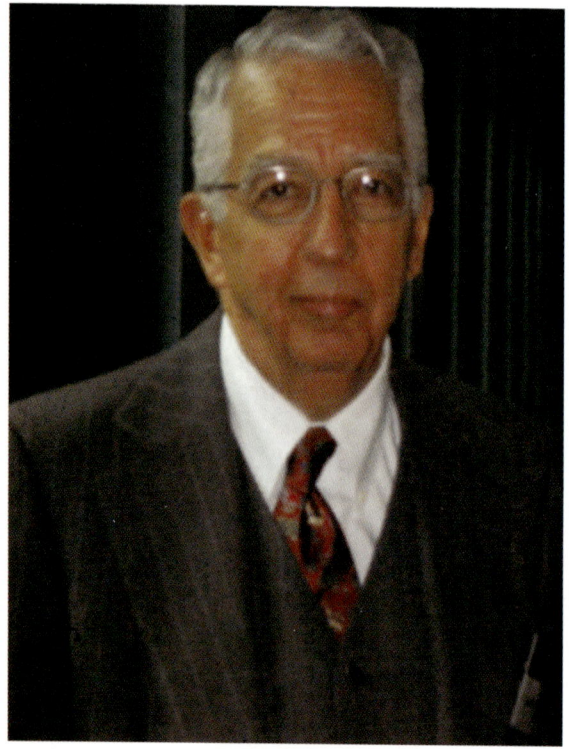

Randall B Griepp

Personal collection

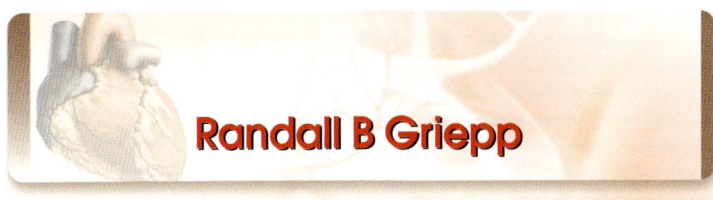

Randall B Griepp

Born   :   1946
Location   :   Mt. Sinai Hospital, New York

Contributions

- The use of deep hypothermia and circulatory arrest for aortic arch aneurysms
- The introduction in USA of the Elephant Trunk Technique for thoraco abdominal aneurysms

Interesting Fact

- Was actively involved in the first heart and lung transplants in the USA

Reference

Griepp RB, Stinson EB, Clark DA, Shumway NE, A two-year experience with human heart transplantation, Calif Med; 1970; 113: 17–26.

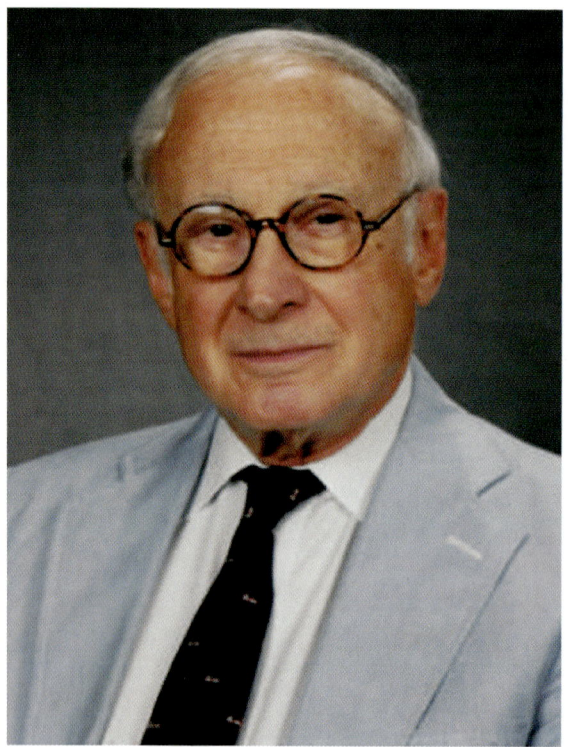

Hermes C Grillo

Reproduced with permission from CTSNet

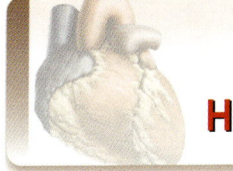

Hermes C Grillo

Dates	:	2nd October, 1923–14th October, 2006
Location	:	Massachusetts General Hospital, Harward University, Boston, USA

Contributions

- Pioneered techniques in Tracheal Surgery
- *Surgery of the Trachea and Bronchi*, is the only textbook on airway surgery

Interesting Facts

- Father of tracheal surgery
- Traveller

Reference

Grillo HC, Bendixen HH, Gerphart T, Resection of the carina and lower trachea, Ann Surg; November 1963; 158(5): 889–893.

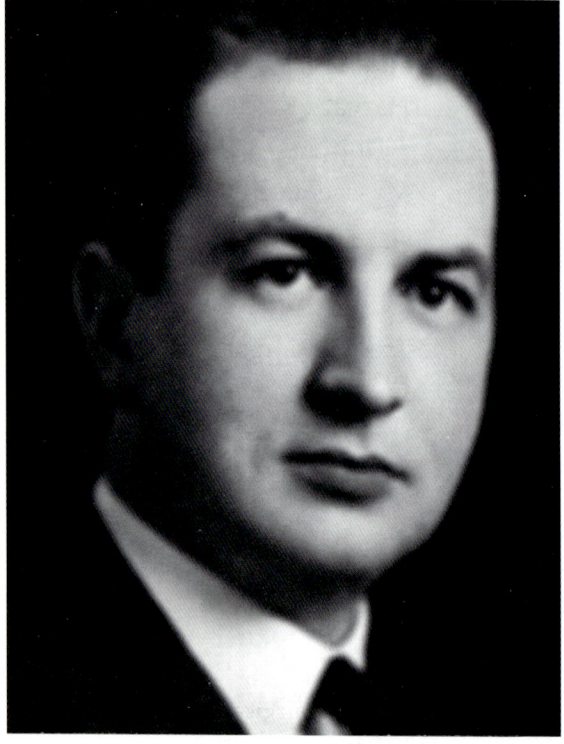

Robert E Gross

Courtesy of Gerald Rainer

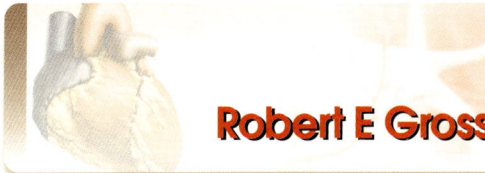

Robert E Gross

Dates   : 2nd July, 1905–11th October, 1988

Location : Harvard Medical School

               Children's Hospital, Boston, Massachusetts, USA

Contributions

- The first successful ligation of patent ductus arteriosus on August 28, 1938.
- The first successful correction of coarctation of aorta in the USA

Interesting Fact

- He was denied permission to do the surgery for PDA interruption

Reference

Gross RE and Hubbard JH, Surgical ligation of a patent ductus arteriosus: Report of first successful case, JAMA 1939; 112: 729–731.

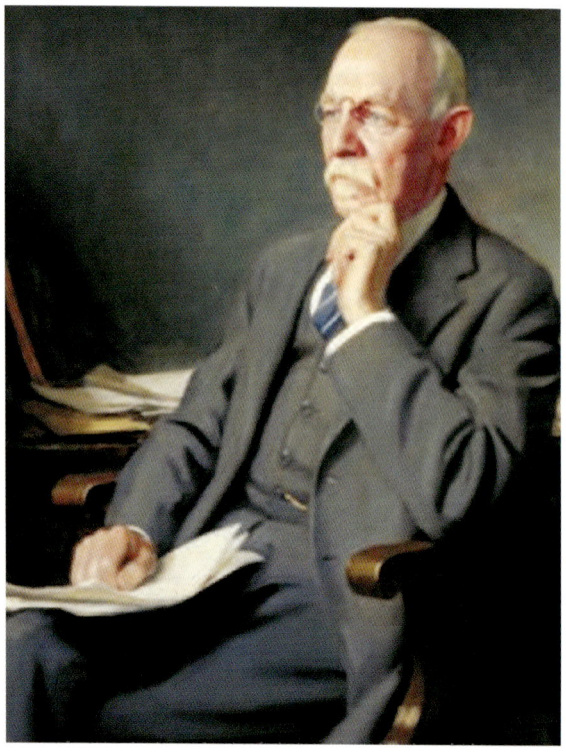

William Stewart Halsted

Courtesy of Dr Duke Cameron, Johns Hopkins University

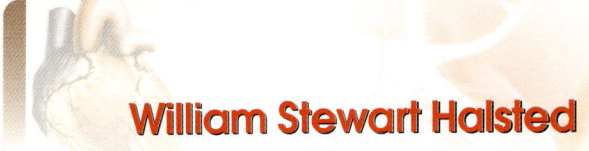

William Stewart Halsted

Dates   : 23rd September, 1852–7th September, 1922

Location : Johns Hopkins University, Baltimore, Maryland, USA

Contributions

- Father of modern surgical techniques
- Introduced rubber gloves and aseptic techniques
- Tenets of Halsted; the basic principles of surgery
- Introduced residency training program
- Halsted radical mastectomy

Interesting Fact

- A great innovator

Reference

Halsted WS, Ligature and suture materials: The employment of fine silk in preference to catgut and the advantages of transfixion of tissues and vessels in control of hemorrhage; Also an account of the introduction of gloves, gutta-percha tissue and silver foil, JAMA 1913; 60: 1119–1126.

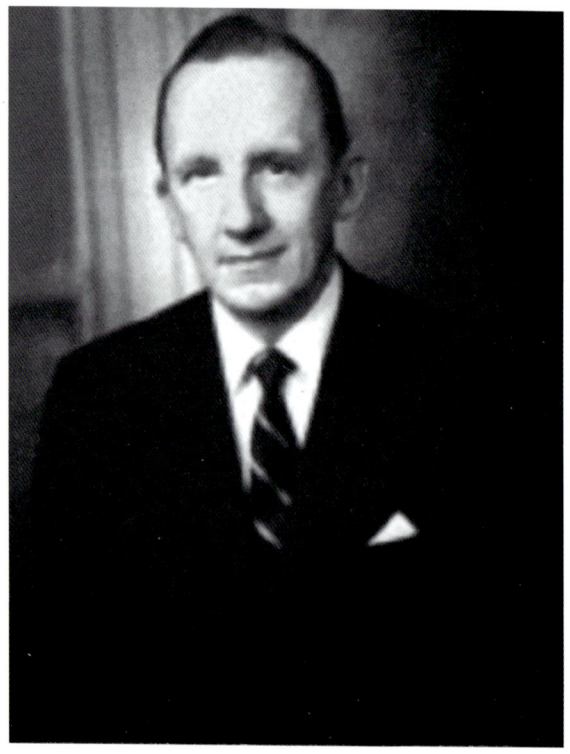

C. Rollins Hanlon

Reproduced with permission from Annals of Thoracic Surgery

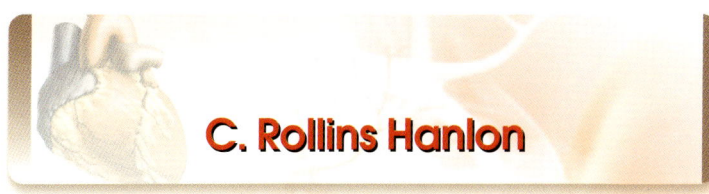

C. Rollins Hanlon

Date of Birth : 8th February, 1915
Location   : Johns Hopkins University, Baltimore
St. Louis University School of Medicine

Contribution

- The creation of a large atrial septal defect for transposition of great arteries in 1950

Interesting Fact

- Along with Dr Mrs Hanlon received the distinguished philanthropist award in 2004 from American College of Surgeons

Reference

Rollins HR and Alfred B, Complete transposition of the aorta and the pulmonary artery. Experimental observations on venous shunts as corrective procedure, Ann Surg 1948; 127: 385–397.

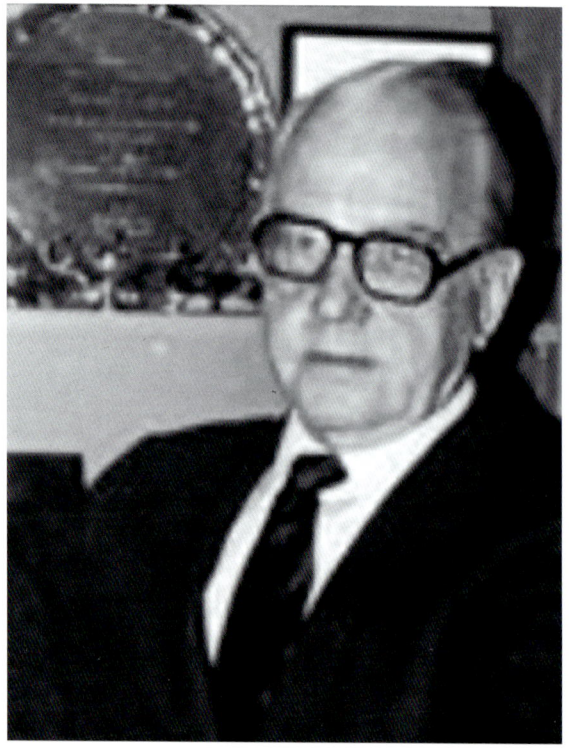

Dwight Emary Harken

Courtesy of Gerald Rainer

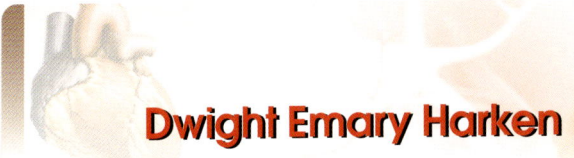

Dwight Emary Harken

Died : Died 29th August, 1993

Location : Brigham and Women's Hospital, Boston Massachusetts, USA

Contributions

- Recognised the need for and developed the concept of intensive care unit in 1951.
- Performed the second successful closed mitral valvotomy in 1948.

Interesting Facts

- He founded "Mended Hearts"—a group that helps patients to overcome stress and anxiety of surgery
- He played major role in the founding of "Heart House" which is headquarters of "The American College of Cardiology"

Reference

Harken DE, Laurence EB, Paul WF, Leona NR, The surgical treatment of mitral stenosis. I. Valvuloplasty, New Engl J Med 1948; 239: 801–809.

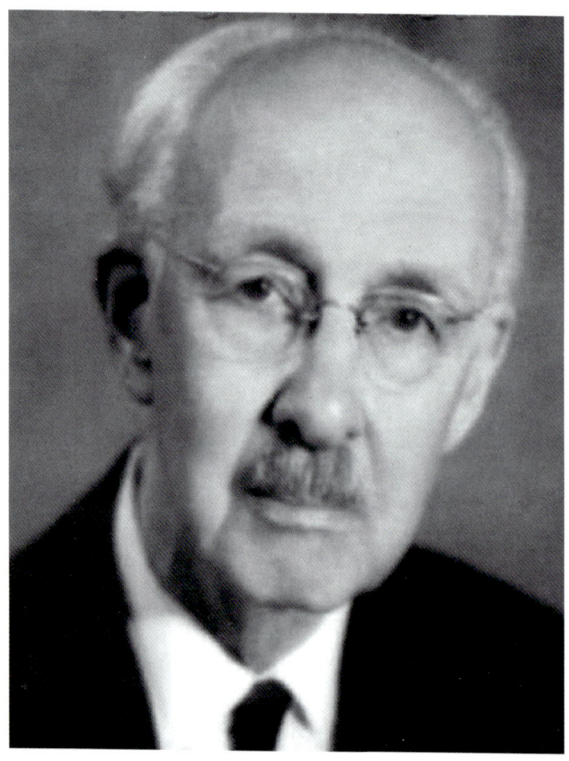

Emile Frederic Holman

Reproduced with permission from Elsevier

Emile Frederic Holman

Dates   : 1890–1977

Location : Stanford University, California, USA

Contributions

- The understanding of arteriovenous fistulae and the pathological effects
- He proposed ligation of patient ductus arteriosus in 1925
- He recommended transplantation of skin from mother to child for burns

Interesting Fact

- He championed the cause for universal understanding among patrons

Reference

Holman EF, Gerbode F, Purdy A, The patent ductus. A review of seventy-five cases with treatment including an aneurysm of the ductus and one of the pulmonary artery, J Thorac Surg 1953; 25: 111–142.

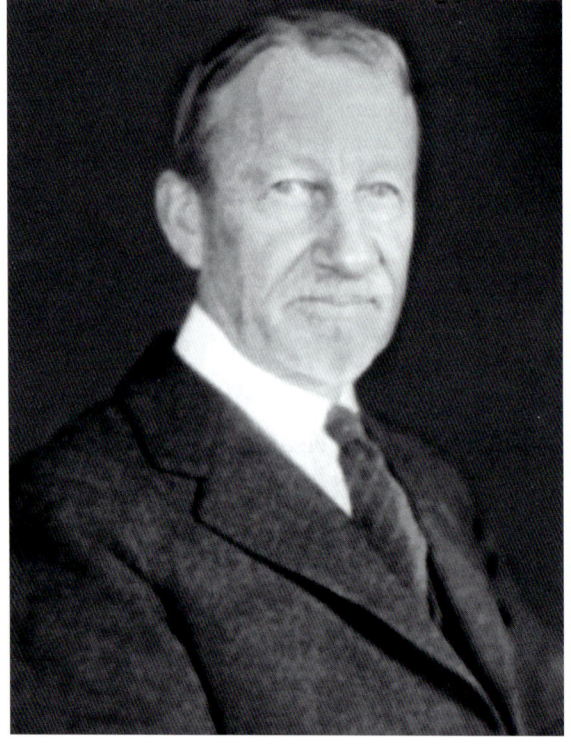

William Henry Howell

Reproduced with permission from Elsevier

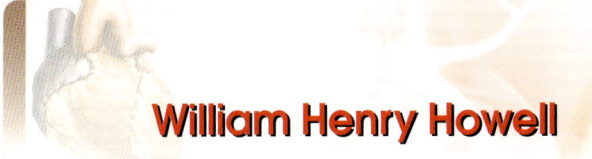

William Henry Howell

Dates : 1860–1945

Location : Johns Hopkins University, Baltimore, Maryland, USA

Contribution

• Together with Mclean discovered and purified Heparin in 1916

Interesting Fact

• It appears that Jay Mclean, a medical student, actually isolated Heparin in Howell's laboratory in 1916

Reference

Howell WH, Holt E, Two new factors in blood coagulation Heparin and pro-antithrombin, Amer. J. Physiol. 1918; 47: 328–341.

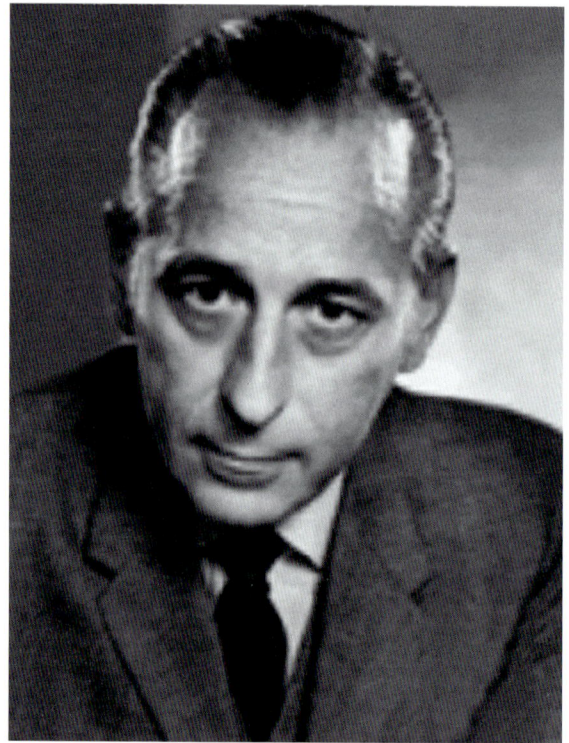

Charles Anthony Hufnagel

Reproduced with permission from CTSNet

Charles Anthony Hufnagel

Dates   : 15th August, 1916–13th May, 1989
Location   : Boston, Massachusetts, USA
              Georgetown, Washington, USA

Contributions

- The first implantable valve to correct aortic regurgitation. The valve was implanted with a sutureless technique in the descending thoracic aorta.
- He made a vascular graft made of Lucite to bridge gaps in arteries.

Interesting Fact

- In 1965 at the age of 49 he received the Mendel Medal from Villanova University, Villanova, Pennsylvania, USA where he got his Bachelor of Science degree

Reference

Hufnagel CA, Harvey P, Rabil PJ, McDermott TF, Surgical correction of aortic insufficiency, Surgery 1954; 35: 673–683.

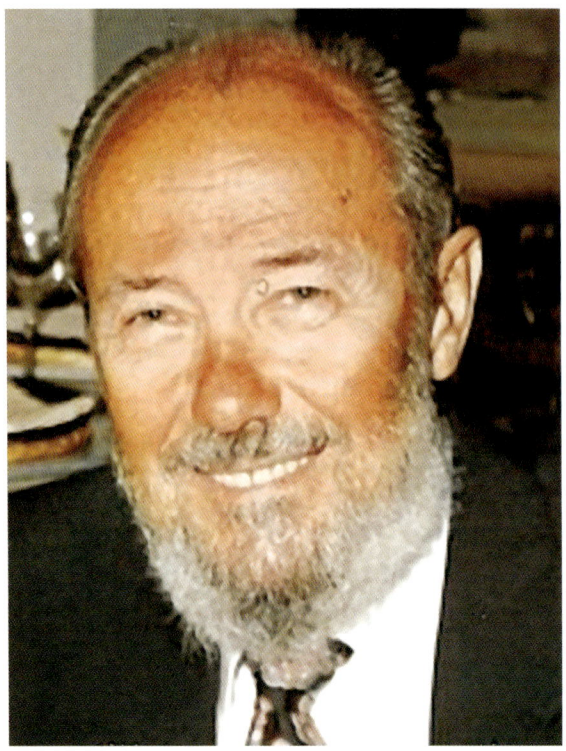

Marian Ion Ionescu

Reproduced with permission from Wikipedia

Marian Ion Ionescu

Born   : 21st August, 1929
Location : Leeds General Infirmary, Leeds, UK

Contributions

- Developed tissue valve prosthesis for heart valve replacement (Ionescu-Shiley valve).
- Surgical instruments—aortic retractors.

Interesting Fact

- Avid mountaineer

Reference

Tandon AP, Smith DR, and Ionescu MI, Sequential Hemodynamic Studies of the Ionescu-Shiley Pericardial Xenograft valve up to six years after implantation, Cardiovasc Dis. September, 1979; 6(3): 271–282.

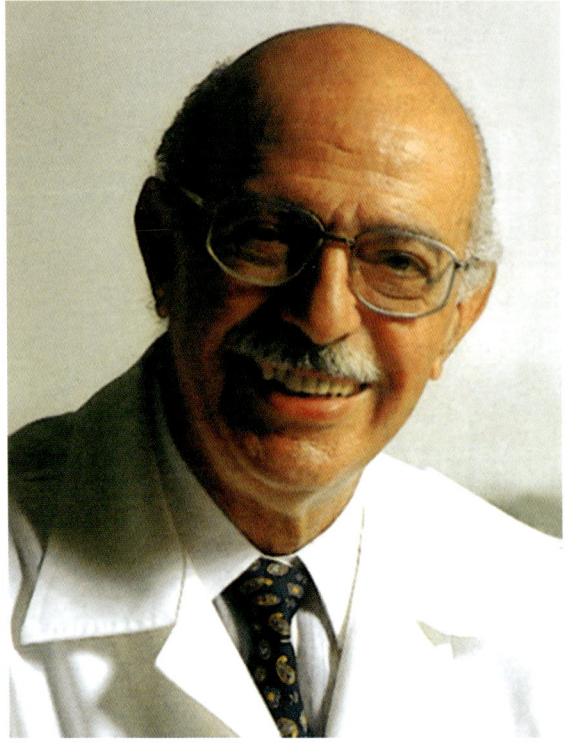

Adib Jatene

Courtesy of GB Pant Hospital

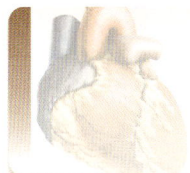

Adib Jatene

Born : 1921

Location : Director, Heart Institute, University of Sao Palo, Brazil

Contributions

- The arterial switch operation for transposition of great arteries
- Started a bioengineering facility and developed a valve prosthesis, bubble oxygenerator and a pacemaker

Interesting Fact

- He was Brazil's Minister for Health from 1992

Reference

Jatene AD, Fontes VF, Paulista PP, de Souza LCB, Neger F, Galantier M, JEMR Souza, Successful anatomic correction of transposition of the great vessels: A preliminary report, Arquivos Brasileiros Cardiologia, 1975; 28: 461.

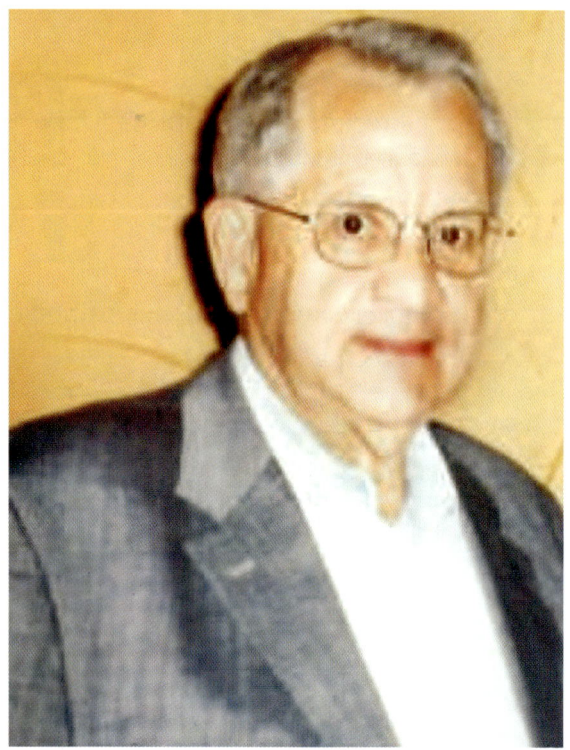

Dudley W Johnson

Personal collection

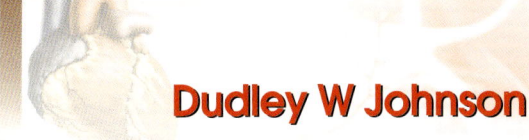

Dudley W Johnson

Date : 4th March, 1930–24th October, 2016

Location : University of Wisconsin, Milwaukee, Wisconsin, USA

Contributions

- Direct coronary artery bypass to the left system
- Coronary endarterectomies

Interesting Fact

- The surgeon for rejects, long bypasses—long endarterectomies

Reference

Johnson DW, Flemma RJ, Lepley D Jr, Ellison EH, Extended treatment of severe coronary artery disease: A total surgical approach, Annals of Surgery 1969; 171: 460–470.

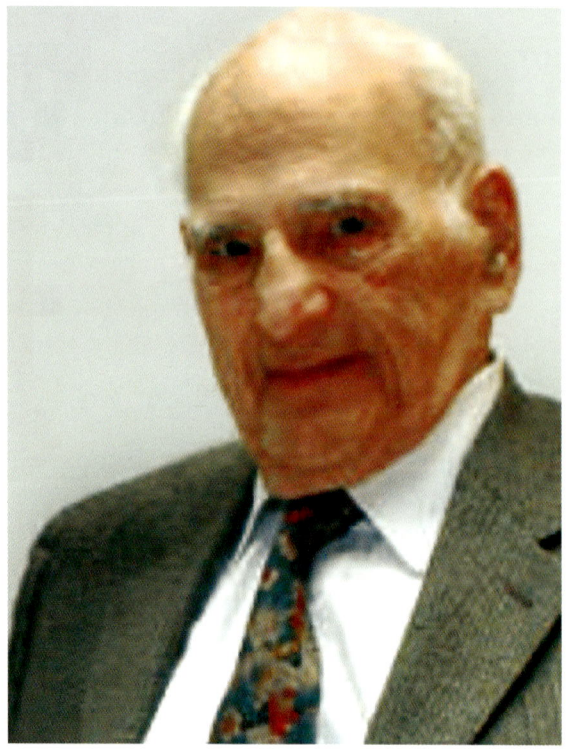

Adrian Kantrowitz

Reproduced with permission From Int. J. Artfi. Organ

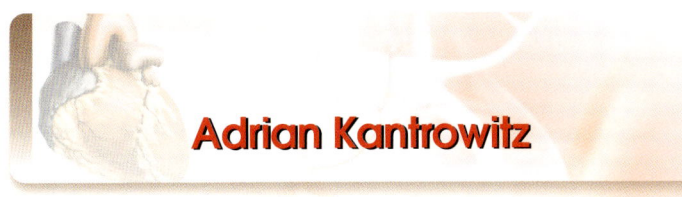

Adrian Kantrowitz

Dates : 4th October, 1918–14th November, 2008

Location : Maimonides Hospital, Brooklyn, New York, USA

Contributions

- World's second and fifth heart transplant
- The first LV assist device implant in 1966
- The introduction of IABP in 1967

Important Fact

- Used to chase and catch field mice at night for experimental work in NY

Reference

Kantrowitz A, Tjonneland S, Freed PS, Philips SJ, Butner AN, Sherman JL, Initial clinical experience with intra-aortic balloon pumping in cardiogenic shock, JAMA, 1968; 203: 135–140.

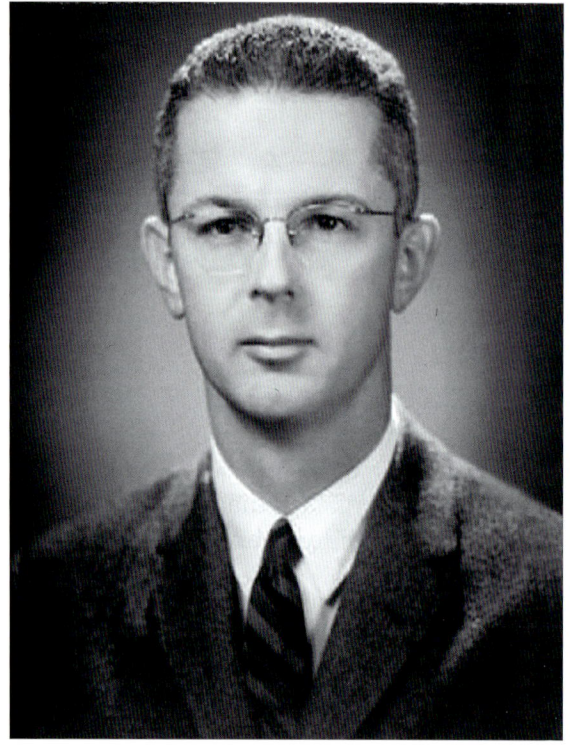

John W Kirklin

Reproduced with permission from Elsevier

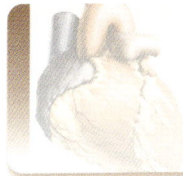

John W Kirklin

Dates : 1917–2004

Location : Mayo Clinic, Rochester, Minneapolis
University of Alabama at Birmingham
Alabama, USA

Contributions

- Refinement of the heart lung machine with IBM which provided the real impetus for open heart surgery
- Technical expertise in the treatment of congenital heart defects, especially tetralogy of Fallot, ventricular septal defects, etc.
- Co-authored textbook "Cardiac Surgery" with Sir Brian Barratt Boyes—considered an authoritative textbook

Interesting Fact

- Was a Neurosurgeon to begin with. Introduced the blue book, his meticulous desire to bring patient care to mathematical precision

Reference

Kirklin JW, DuShane JW, Patrick RT, Donald DE, Hetzel PS, Harshbarger HG, Wood EH, Intracardiac surgery with the aid of a mechanical pump oxygenator system (Gibbon Type): Report of eight cases, Mayo Clinic Proceedings, 1955; 30: 201–206.

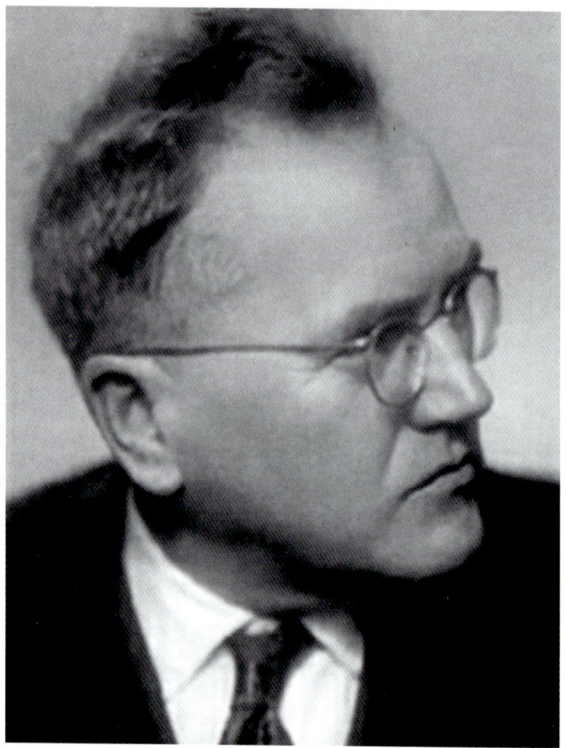

Vasili Kolesov

Reproduced with permission from Texas Heart Institute Journal

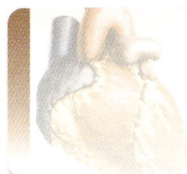

Vasili Kolesov

Dates : 24th September, 1904–1st August, 1992

Location : Leningrad, Russia and USA

Contributions

- The first direct coronary artery internal mammary artery bypass by suture technique, 1961
- The first off pump CABG
- The first use of a intravascular device for continuous coronary perfusion during anesthesia
- The first stapling device for vascular anastomosis
- The first demonstration of long-term patency

Interesting Fact

- Withstood the German siege of Leningrad for 900 days as an army surgeon during World War II

Reference

Kolesov V, Mammary artery—coronary artery anastomosis as a method of treatment for angina pectoris, J Thorac Cardiovasc Surg, 1967; 54: 535–544.

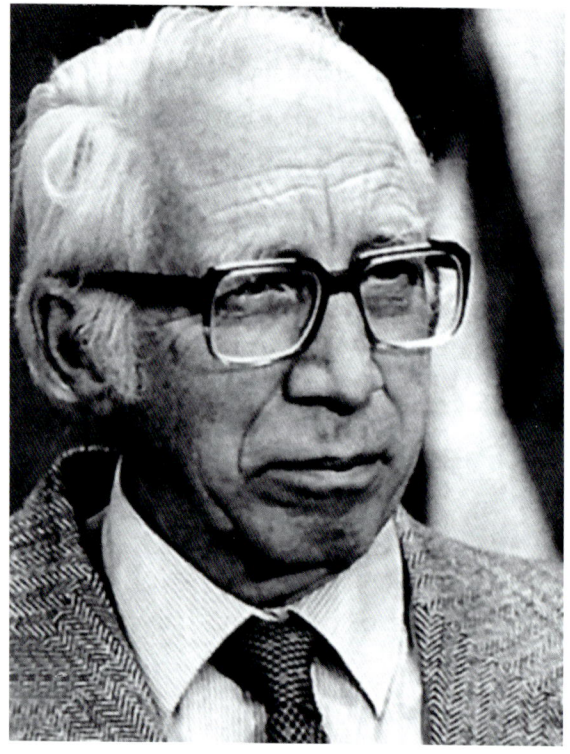

Willem Johan Kolff

Reproduced with permission from Texas Heart Institute Journal

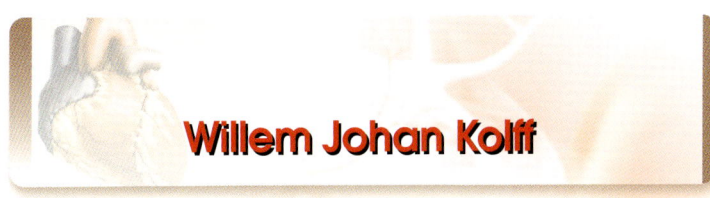

Willem Johan Kolff

Date of Birth : 14th February, 1911–11th Feb, 2009
Location : Kempen-Leiden Germany
Cleveland Clinic, Cleveland OH, USA

Contributions

- In 1943 in Kempen, Germany developed the first artificial kidney
- In 1957 developed the first artificial heart implanted in a dog
- Made a heart lung machine in 1956

Interesting Facts

- Founded the first human blood bank in Europe
- The membrane oxygenator originated from his innovation

Reference

DeVries WC, Anderson JL, Joyce LD, Anderson FL, Hammond EH, Jarvik RK, Kolf WJ, Clinical use of total artificial heart, NEJM 1984; 310: 273–278.

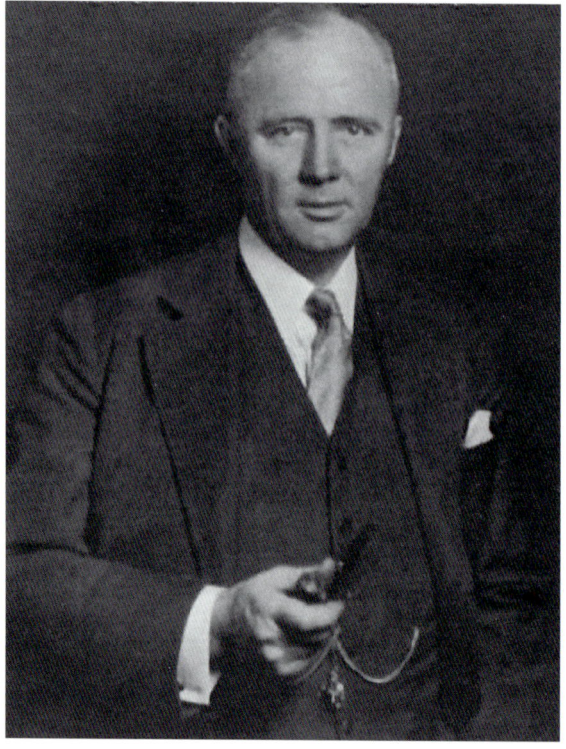

William Bennett Kouwenhoven

Courtesy of Dr Duke Cameron, Johns Hopkins University

William Bennett Kouwenhoven

Dates : 1886–1975

Location : Karlsruhe, Baden, Germany

Johns Hopkins Hospital , USA (Prof of Electrical Engineering, Dean, School of Engineering)

Lecturer in Surgery at Johns Hopkins School of Medicine

Contributions

- The external defibrillator 1957
- The importance of closed chest cardiac massage

Interesting Fact

- He received the first honorary doctorate from Johns Hopkins University in 1964, perhaps the first engineer/ doctor

Reference

Kouwenhoven WB, The development of the defibrillator, Ann Intern Med. September 1969; 71(3): 449–458.

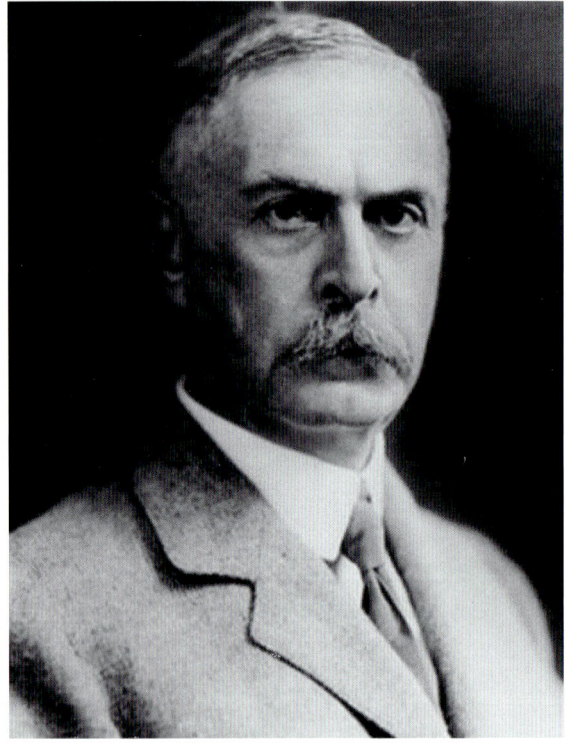

Karl Landsteiner

Internet/Wikipedia

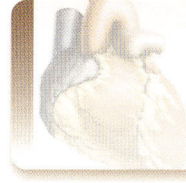

Karl Landsteiner

Dates : 14th June, 1869–26th June, 1943

Location : University of Vienna, Austria
Rockefeller Institute, NY, USA

Contributions

- The discovery of blood groups along with Weiner
- The basics of immunology and the discovery of haptens
- The discovery of Rh factor

Interesting Fact

- Received Nobel Prize for medicine, 1930

Reference

Landsteiner K and Weiner AS, Studies on an agglutinogen (Rh) in human blood reacting with anti-rhesus sera and with human isoantibodies, J Exp Med, September 1941; 74(4): 309–320.

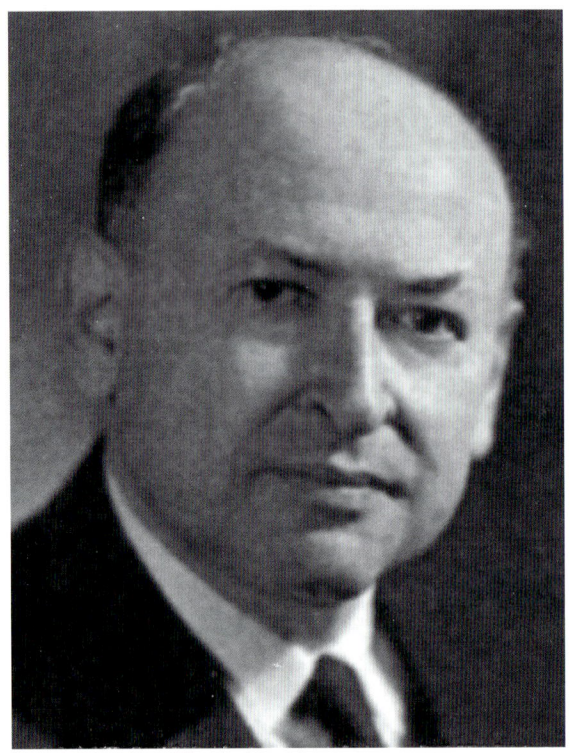

Maurice Lev

Reproduced with permission from Elsevier

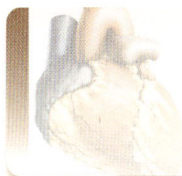

Maurice Lev

Dates	:	13th November 1908–1994
Location	:	University of Illinois, Chicago, USA

Contributions

- The description of conduction system in various congenital anomalies like, VSD, AVSD, CTGA, etc.
- The classification of congenital heart disease along with Saroja Bharti

Interesting Facts

- As a pathologist has taught cardiologists and surgeons
- Obtained a M.Phil at the age of 58

Reference

Lev M and Saphir O, Endophlebohypertrophy and Phlebosclerosis: II. The External and Common Iliac Veins, Am J Pathol, 1952; 28(3): 401–411.

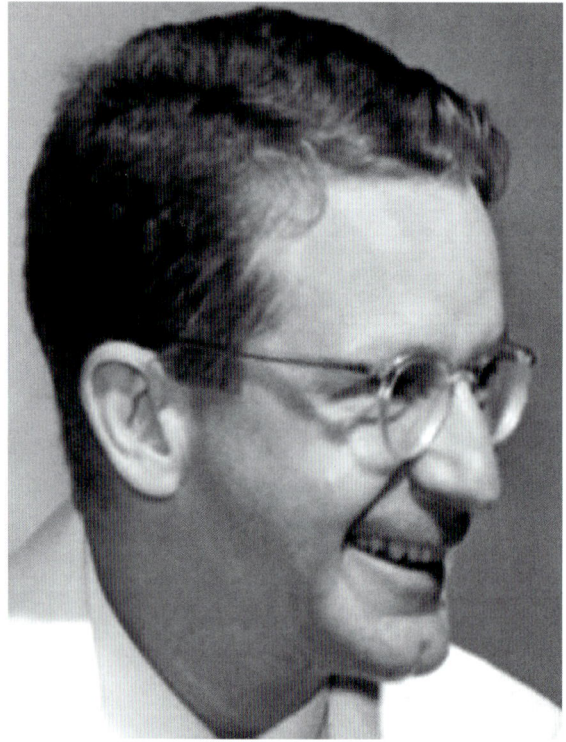

F John Lewis

Reproduced with permission from Annals of Thoracic Surgery

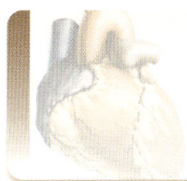

F John Lewis

Dates   : 1916–20th September, 1993
Location : Stanford University, California
              Northwestern University, Chicago

Contribution

• First successful direct vision open heart operation to close an atrial septal defect under hypothermia and inflow occlusion in Minneapolis, Minnesota, September 2, 1952

Interesting Fact

• He wrote monographs on bicycling, hiking and mountaineering. He would do surgery by anesthetising the patient himself.

Reference

Lewis JW and Taufic M, Closure of atrial septal defects with the aid of hypothermia. Experimental accomplishments and the report of one successful case, Surgery, 1953; 33: 52–59.

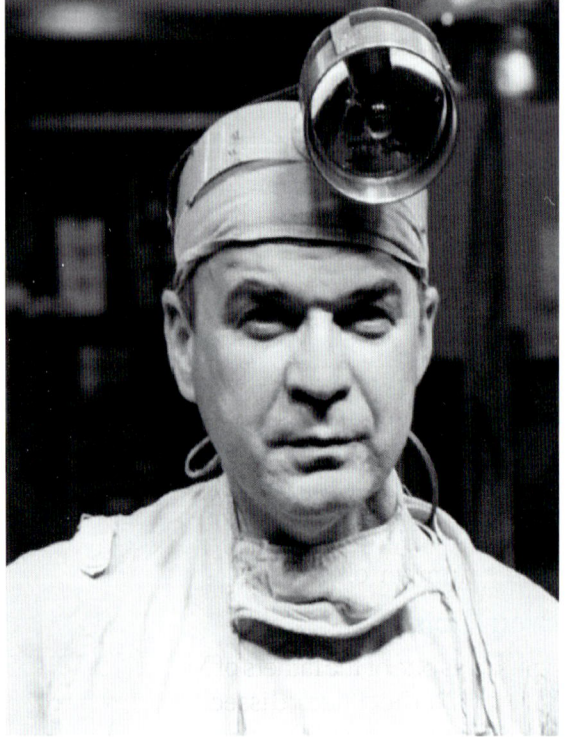

Clarence Walton Lillehei

Courtesy of Dr Kenneth Liao, University of Minnesota

Clarence Walton Lillehei

Dates   : 1918–1999
Location : University of Minnesota, Minneapolis, USA

Contributions

- In 1954 first successful direct vision intracardiac repair with controlled cross circulation for (1) VSD (2) TOF (3) ASD (4) mitral valve repair
- The first successful resuscitation of the heart by electrical stimulation using of transistorised external device. The birth of pacemaker technology
- The development of bubble oxygenator and successful application of open heart procedures using HLM
- The design and development of two heart valves
- The birth of two industrial giants—St. Jude Medical and Medtronic
- Trained a number of pioneers

Interesting Facts

- Recognised as one of the fathers of Modern Cardiac Surgery
- Underwent Radical neck dissection for lymposarcoma of the salivary gland at the age of 30
- MD in physiology and PhD in Surgery

Reference

Lillehei WC, Cohen M, Warden HE, Zeigler NR, Varco RL, The results of direct vision closure of ventricular septal defects in eight patients by means of controlled cross circulation, Surg, Gynaecol Obstet, 1955; 101: 446–466.

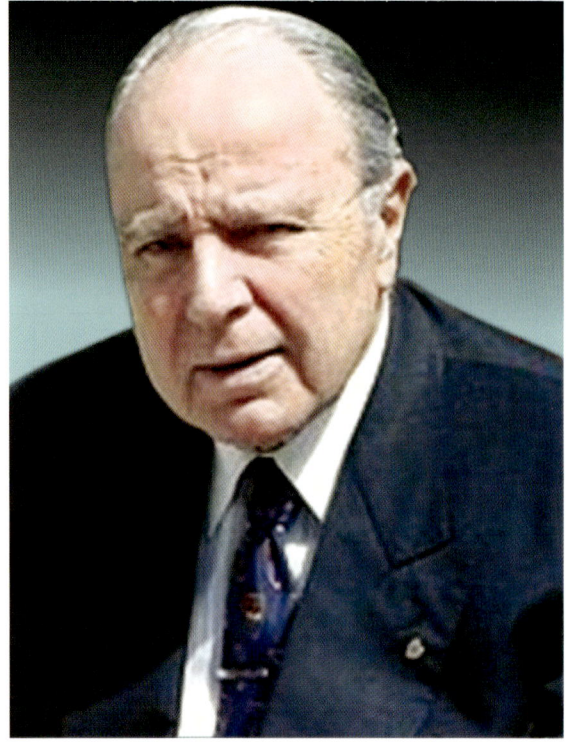

Domingo Liotta

Internet/Wikipedia

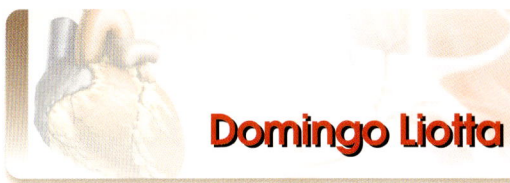

Domingo Liotta

Date of Birth : 29th November, 1924

Location : National University of Cordoba, Argentina
Baylor College, Houston, Texas, USA

Contributions

- Developed the first artificial ventricular assist device for cardiogenic shock, 1963
- Developed the first implantable total artificial heart which was successfully implanted in Man in 1966

Interesting Fact

- Developed a diagnostic technique for carcinoma ampulla of vater and pancreas in 1955

Reference

Liotta D, Hall CW, Henly WS, Cooley DA, Crawford ES, DeBakey ME, Prolonged assisted circulation during and after cardiac or aortic surgery. Prolonged partial left ventricular bypass by means of intracorporeal circulation, Am J Cardiol, 1963; 12: 399–405.

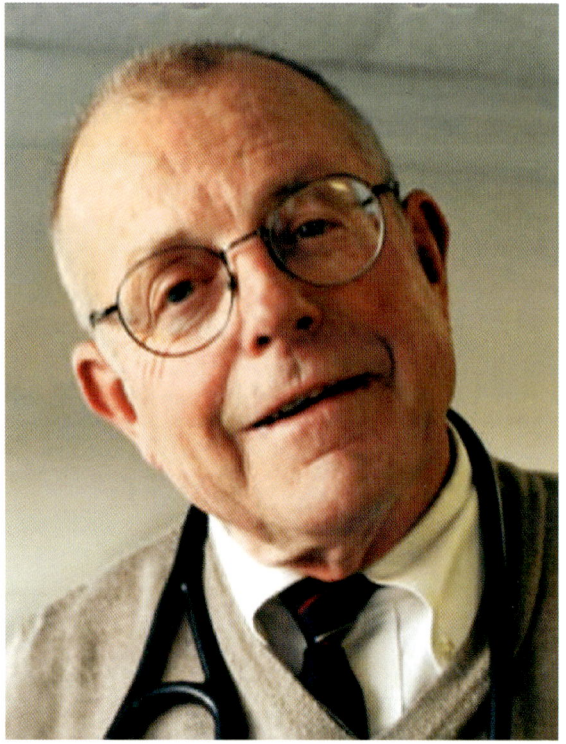

Richard Rowland Lower

Reproduced with permission from Elsevier

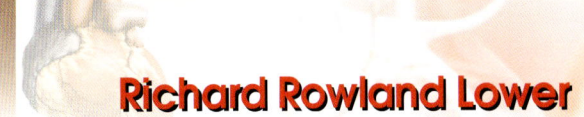

Richard Rowland Lower

Dates : 15th August, 1929–17th May, 2008

Location : Stanford University, San Francisco, California, USA

University of Virginia, Richmond, Virginia, USA

Contributions

- The technique of orthotopic heart transplantation along with Norman Shumway
- Performed the 3rd transplant at University of Virginia

Interesting Facts

- Was sued by the family of an organ donor
- Worked as family physician for the poor at Richmond, Virginia

Reference

Lower RR and Shumway NE, Studies on orthotopic homotransplantations of the canine heart, Surgical Forum, 1960; 11: 18–19.

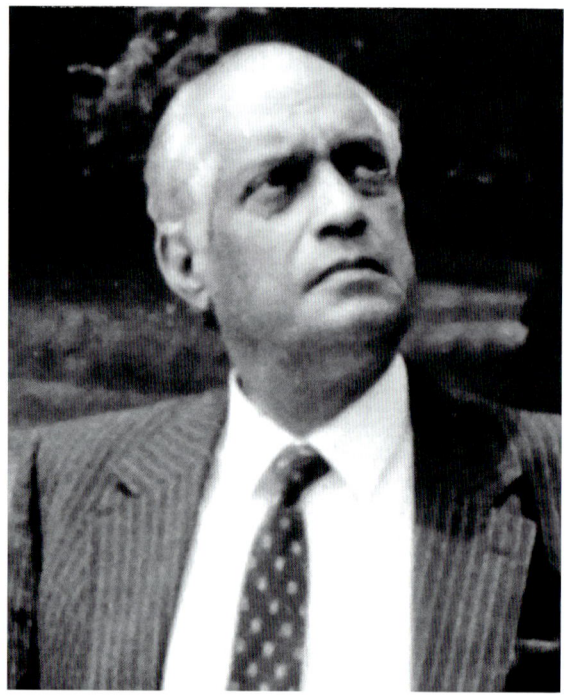

Gerard (Gerry)
Martin Mascarenhas

Gerard (Gerry) Martin Mascarenhas

Dates : 1925–1999

Location : SDS Sanatorium, Bangalore Medical College

Dean, St. John's Medical College Bengaluru

Contributions

- Trained with Andrew Logan in Edinburgh and Frank Spencer in Lexington, Kentucky, USA.
- Developed and established the first cardiothoracic department in Bengaluru. Worked in Government hospitals to serve the poor.
- Received Gold medal for his contribution to cardiac surgery from Government of Karnataka.

Interesting Facts

- Maverick surgeon who was a one-man team. He anesthetised, intubated, positioned, operated and cared for his patients.
- Best papa for his children.

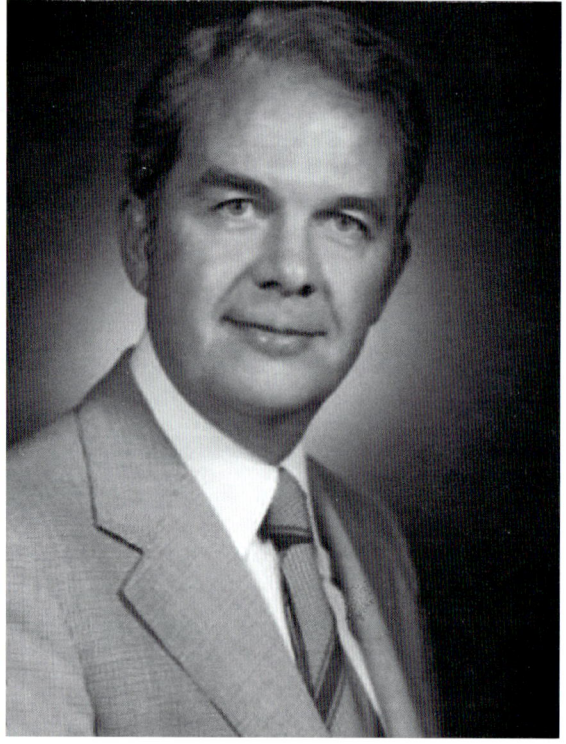

Dwight Charles McGoon

Reproduced with permission from Mayo Clinic

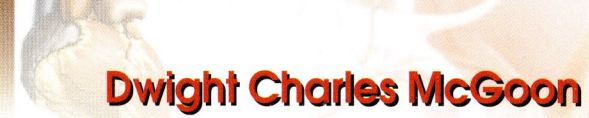

Dwight Charles McGoon

Born : 1925

Location : Johns Hopkins University, MD

Mayo Clinic Rochester, Minnesota, USA

Contributions

- The first successful correction of truncus arteriosus
- Mitral valve repair for prolapsed AML
- Edited the Journal of Thoracic and Cardiovascular Surgery

Interesting Fact

- Considered surgeon "of the impossible"

Reference

McGoon DC, Manin HT, Vlad P, Kirklin JW, The surgical treatment of supravalvular aortic stenosis. J Thorac Cardiovasc Surg 1961; 41: 125–133.

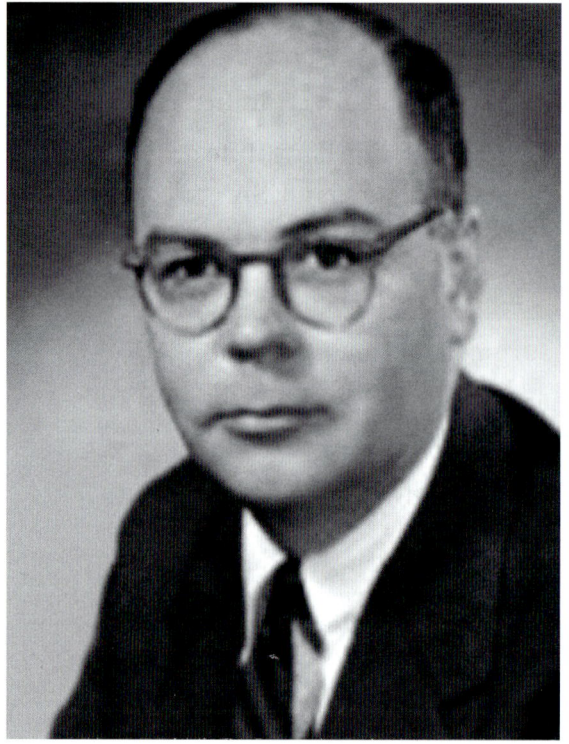

Andrew Glenn Morrow

Reproduced with permission from Annals of Thoracic Surgery

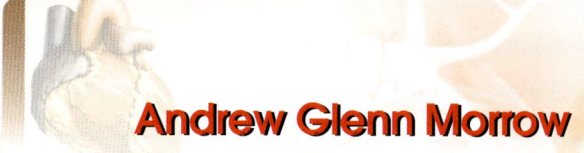

Andrew Glenn Morrow

Dates : 1922–1982

Location : National Heart Institute

National Institute of Health, Bethesda, Maryland, USA

Contribution

• The surgical treatment of idiopathic hypertrophic subaortic stenosis (IHSS) by septal myomectomy

Interesting Fact

• He was diagnosed to have IHSS

Reference

Morrow AG and Brockenbrough EC, Surgical Treatment of Idiopathic Hypertrophic Subaortic Stenosis: Technic and Hemodynamic Results of Subaortic Ventriculotomy, Ann Surg, August 1961; 154(2): 181–189.

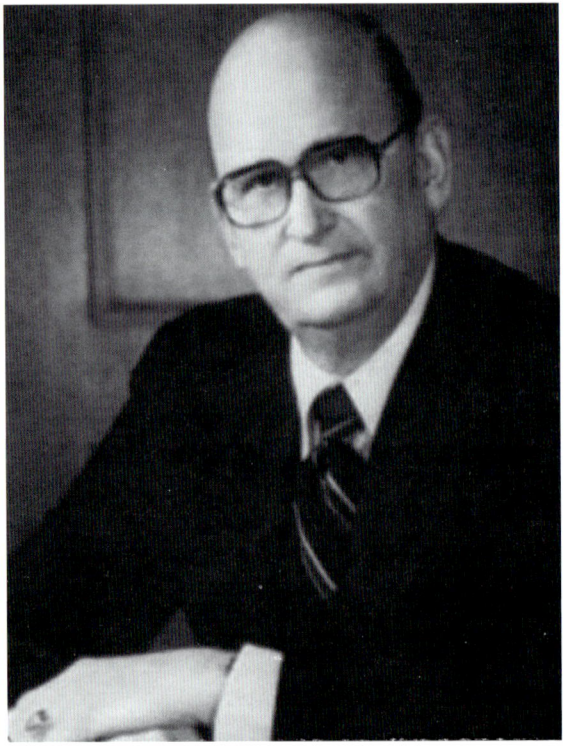

William H Muller

Reproduced with permission from Annals of Thoracic Surgery

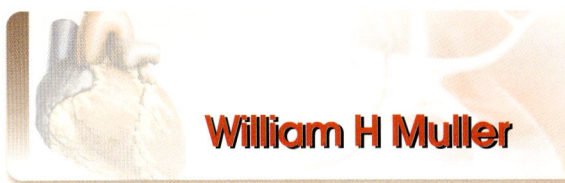

William H Muller

Born : 19th August, 1919

Location : University of California at Los Angeles
University of Virginia School of Medicine
at Charlottsville

Contribution

- Along with Damman classified ventricular septal defects and introduced the concept and techniques of pulmonary artery banding

Interesting Fact

- He is a master craftsman and has built most of the furniture at his residence

Reference

Muller WH, The surgical treatment of the transposition of the pulmonary veins, Annals of Surgery, 1951; 134: 683–693.

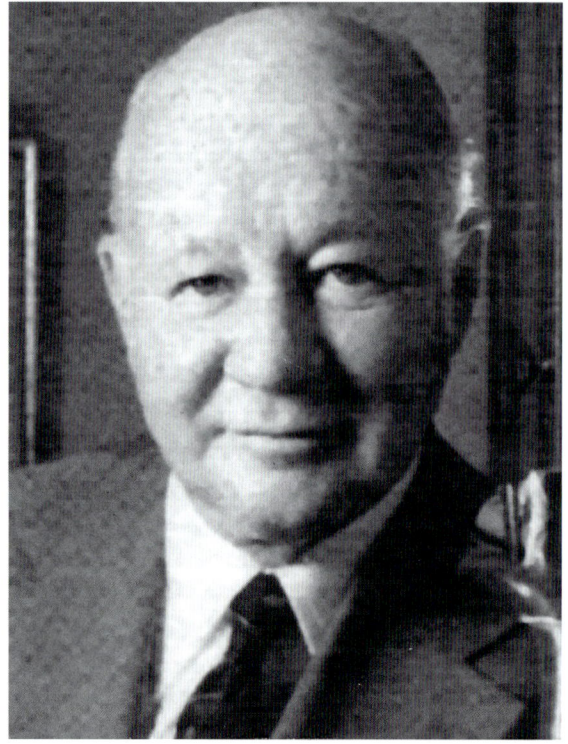

William Thorton Mustard

Courtesy of Dr Gerald Rainer

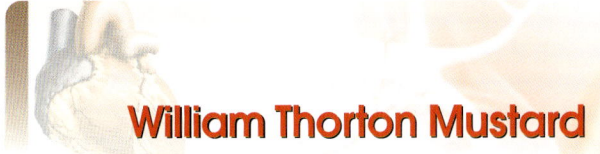

William Thorton Mustard

Dates : 8th August, 1914–11th December, 1987

Location : Hospital for Sick Children, Toronto, Canada

Contributions

- The Mustard Procedure for transposition of great arteries
- First to perform open heart surgery using a mechanical pump and biological lung in a dog at the Banting Institute

Interesting Facts

- Decorated with an MBE (Member of the British Empire)
- A Mustard operation for use of the hip in patients with polio was devised by him

Reference

Mustard WT, Successful two-stage correction of transposition of the great vessels, Surgery 1964; 55: 469–472.

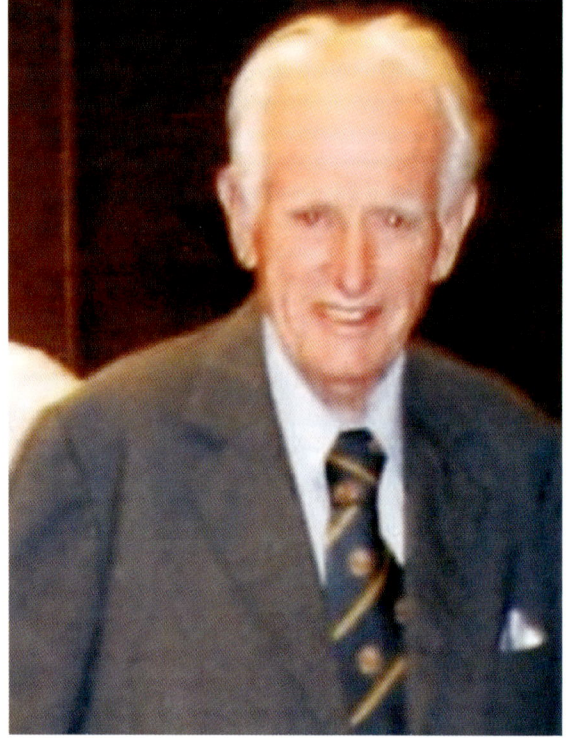

Rowan Nicks

Personal collection

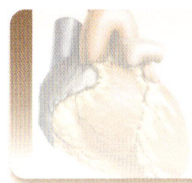

Rowan Nicks

Dates   : 24th Feb, 1914–26th May, 2011
Location   : University of Sydney, Australia

Contributions

- The design of pacemaker for automatic control of heart rate (demand pacemaking)
- The technique of aortic root enlargement for AVR

Interesting Fact

- Travelled extensively around the world training surgeons in India, Africa, Asia Pacific regions

Reference

Nicks R, Cartmill T, Bernstein L, Hypoplasia of the aortic root: The problem of aortic valve replacement. Thorax, May 1970; 25(3): 339–346.

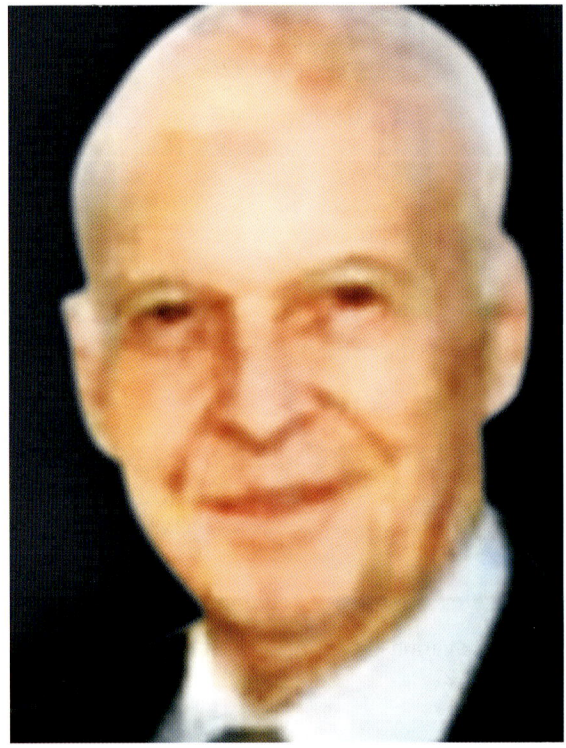

Victor Parsonnet

Reproduced with permission from CTSNet

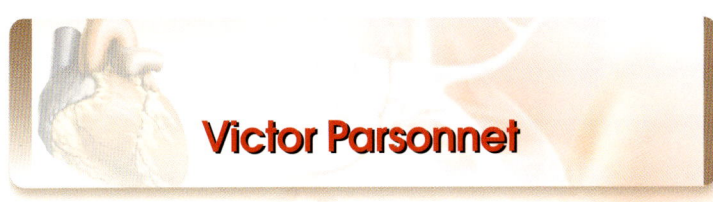

Victor Parsonnet

Dates   :   29th August, 1924–21st April, 2002

Location   :   Newark Beth Israel Hospital, Newark,
New Jersey (USA)

Contributions

- The physiology and technology of pacemaking and pacemakers
- Development of large heart transplant program

Interesting Facts

- Was the Chairman of New Jersey Sympony Orchestra
- Was an accomplished pianist

Reference

Parsonnet V, Innovations in cardiac pacemakers–1975, Cardiac vasc Dis, 1976; 3(1): 11–21.

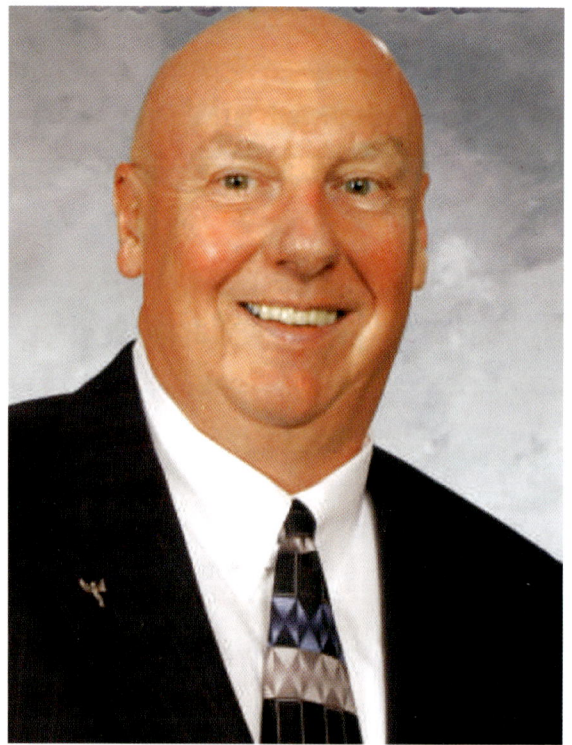

Willis J Potts

Reproduced with permission from Elsevier

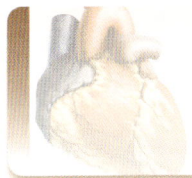

Willis J Potts

Dates   : 1895–1968

Location   : Rush Medical College, University of Chicago, USA

Professor, Northwestern University, Chicago, USA

Contributions

- The Potts' shunt—descending aorta to left pulmonary artery 1946
- The Potts' clamp which partially occludes the aorta

Interesting Fact

- He had a great sense of humour

Reference

Potts WJ, Smith S, Gibson S, Anastomosis of the aorta to a pulmonary artery; certain types in congenital heart disease, JAMA, November 1946; 132(11): 627–631.

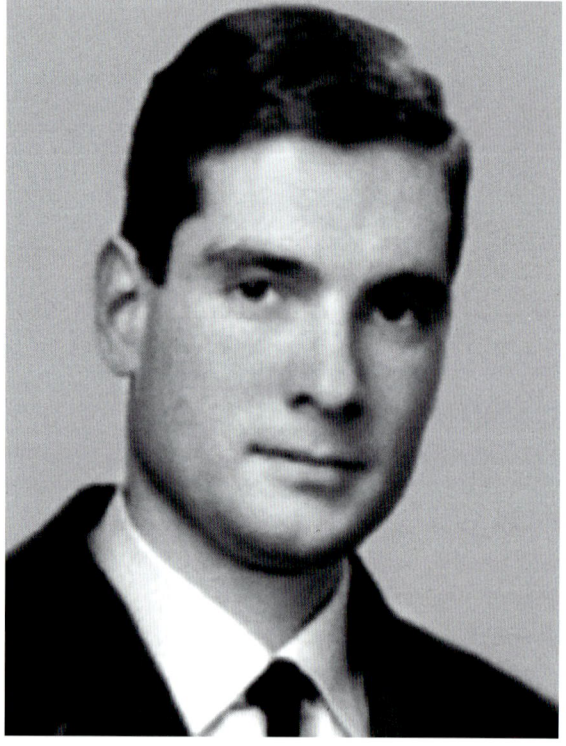

Giancarlo Rastelli

Reproduced with permission from Annals of Thoracic Surgery

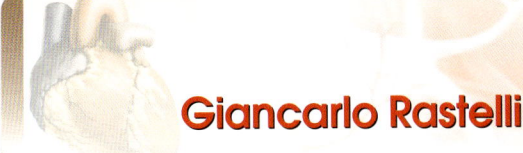

Giancarlo Rastelli

Dates : 25th June, 1933 – January, 1970

Location : Mayo clinic, Rochester, Minnesota, US

Contributions

- The classification of AV canal defects
- The Rastelli operation for TGA/VSD and truncus arteriosus

Interesting Fact

- Died young (37 years) of Hodgkin's lymphoma

Reference

Rastelli GC, A new approach to "Anatomic" repair of transposition of the great arteries. Mayo clinic proceedings, 1969; 44: 12.

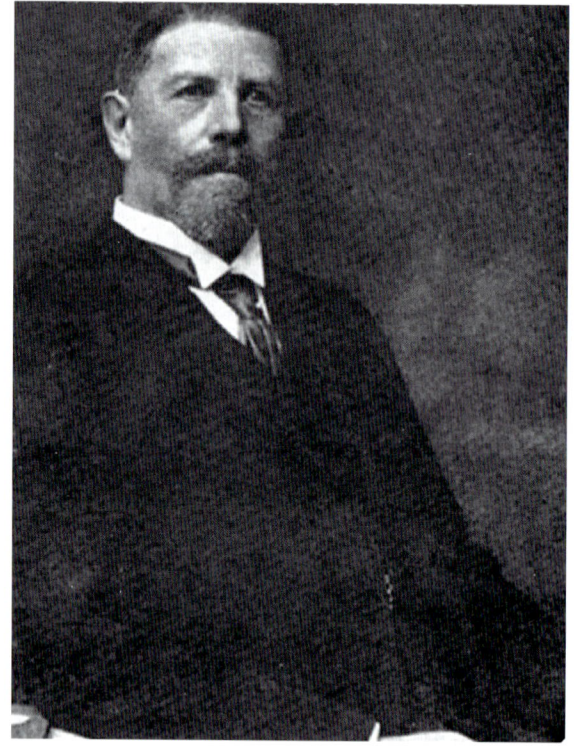

Ludwig Wilhelm Carl Rehn

Reproduced with permission from Elsevier

Ludwig Wilhelm Carl Rehn

Dates : 13th April, 1849–29th May, 1930

Location : Head of Surgery–Stradir–Kraken, Frankfurt, Germany

Contributions

• On 9th September, 1896 he successfully sutured a wound in the heart clearly the beginning of surgery on the human heart

Interesting Fact

• First thyroidectomy for Goitre in 1880 and described carcinoma of the bladder in Aniline dye workers

Reference

Rehn LWC, On penetrating cardiac injuries and cardiac suturing, Archiv Fuersche Chirugie, 1897; 55: 315–329.

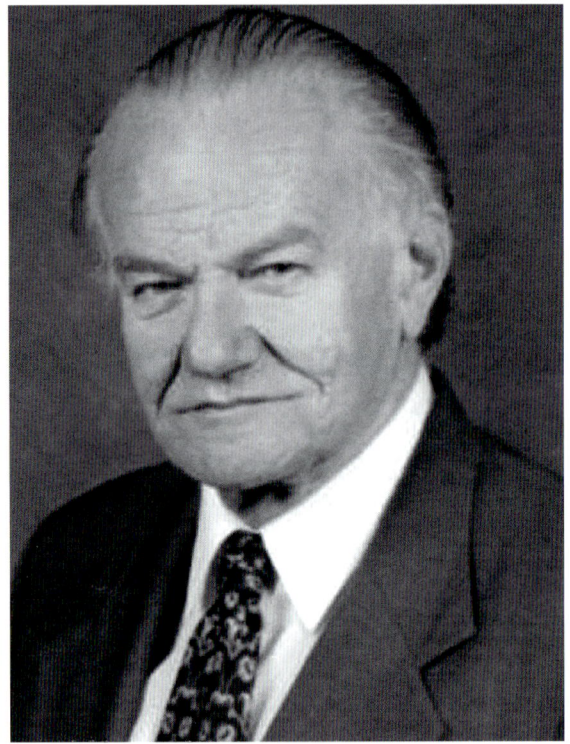

Francis Robicsek

Reproduced with Permission from CTSNet

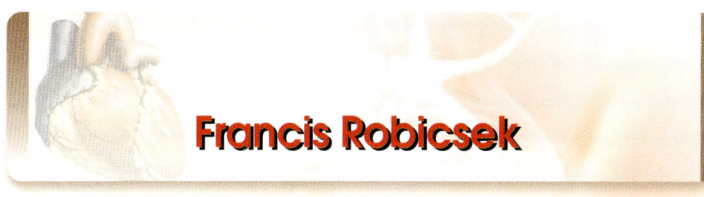

Francis Robicsek

Born   : 4th July, 1925

Location   : Prof of Surgery, University of North
                   Carolina

Contribution

• The surgical correction of pectus excavatum.

Interesting Fact

• Prof of Anthropology and Biomedical engineering.

Reference

Robicsek F, Sanger PW, Taylor FH, Daugherty H, Peripheral Stricture of the Pulmonary Artery Treated by Cava-Pulmonary Anastomosis, Annals of Surg, Dec 1964; 160(6): 1066–1068.

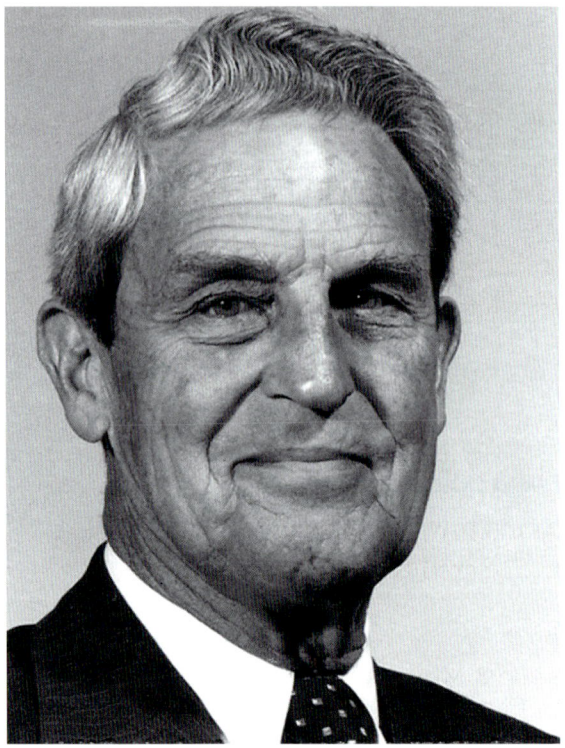

Benson B Roe

Reproduced with permission from CTSNet

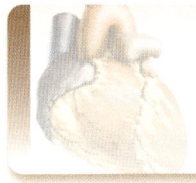

Benson B Roe

Dates	:	1918–6th August, 2012
Location	:	University of California of San Francisco (UCSF) San Francisco, California, USA

Contributions

- One of the persons to introduce cardioplegia
- Aided in the development of thoracic surgery as a speciality

Interesting Facts

- Champion rowing team member
- Worked to eradicate narcotic drug abuse

Reference

Roe BB, Kelly PB, Myers JL, Moore DW, Tricuspid leaflet aortic valve prosthesis, Circulation 1966; 33 (suppl 1): 124–130.

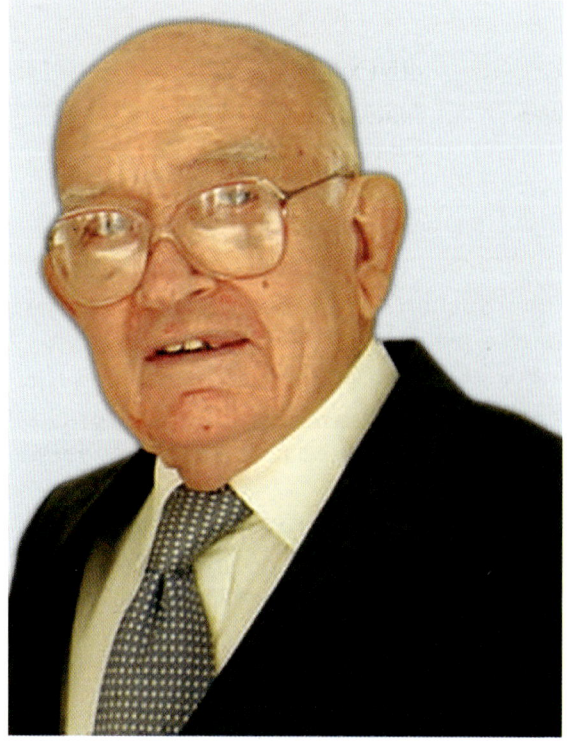

Donald Nixon Ross

Personal Collection

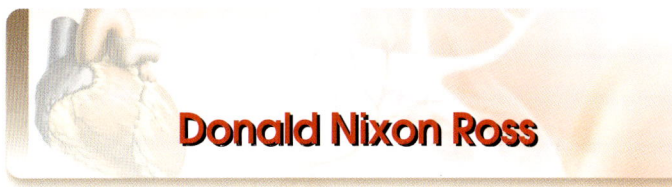

Donald Nixon Ross

Date of Birth : 4th October, 1922–7th July, 2014

Location : National Heart Hospital, London, England

Contributions

- The introduction of the pulmonary autograft as a living substitute for diseased aortic and mitral valves—the Ross operations
- The introduction of the aortic homograft as a replacement for diseased aortic valves in the scalloped subcoronary technique

Interesting Fact

- For two decades Dr. Ross was the only surgeon who believed in and performed the Ross procedure.

Reference

Ross DN, Homograft replacement of the aortic valve, Lancet 1962; 2: 487.

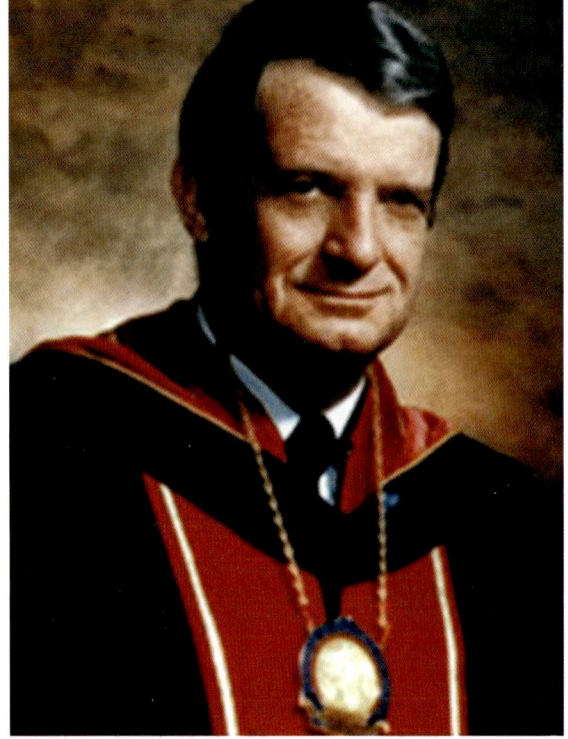

David C Sabiston

Reproduced with permission from CTSNet

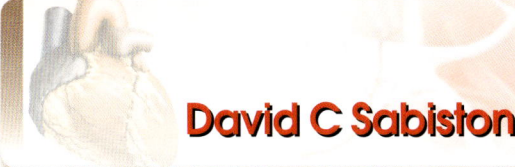

David C Sabiston

Born : 1924

Location : Duke University, Durham, North California, USA

Contribution

• The understanding of coronary circulation

Interesting Facts

• Alumnus of Johns Hopkins and the hospital for sick children
• Edited one of the first textbooks on Thoracic Surgery

Reference

Sabiston DC, Neill CA, Taussig HB, The direction of flow in anomalous left coronary artery arising from the pulmonary artery, Circulation, 1960; 22: 591–597.

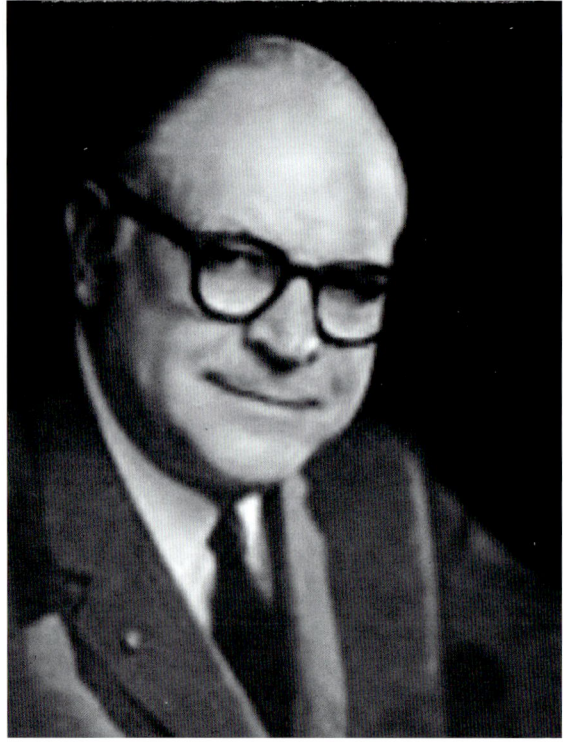

Paul C Samson

Courtesy of Gerald Rainer

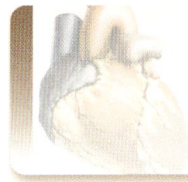

Paul C Samson

Dates : 1905–1982
Location : Oakland, CA, USA

Contributions
- The treatment of empyema thoracis
- The management of war injuries

Interesting Facts
- A giant in stature at 6 ft 6 in
- Was in the US Olympic water polo team
- First President of The Society of Thoracic Surgeons

Reference
Burford TH, Parker ED, Samson PC, Early pulmonary decortication in the treatment of post-traumatic empyema, Ann Surg, August 1945; 122(2); 163–190.

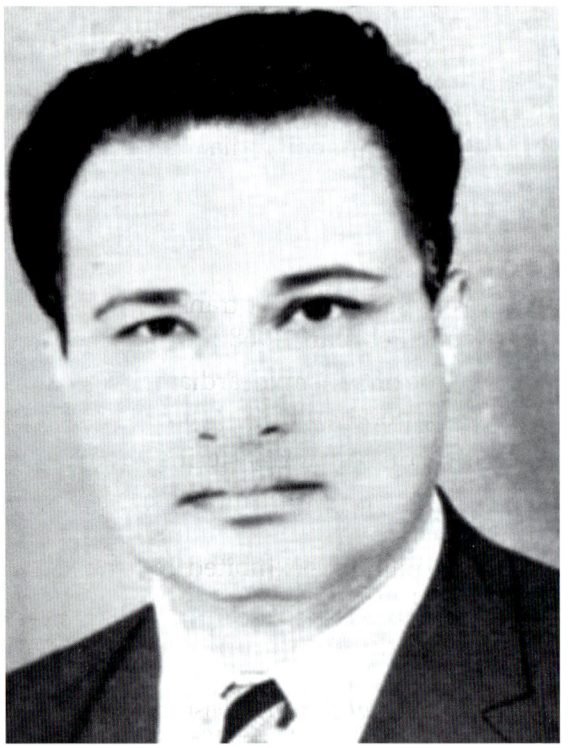

Profulla Kumar Sen

Permission from IJTCVS

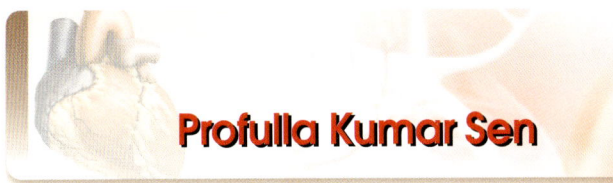

Profulla Kumar Sen

Dates	:	7th December, 1915–22nd July, 1982
Location	:	King Edward Memorial Hospital, Mumbai, India

Contributions

- The first and second heart transplants in India (6th in the world) in February 1968
- The technique of transmyocardial revascularisation (the snake heart operation)
- The description of "Aortoarteritis"

Interesting Fact

- A poet and painter—exhibited his paintings in India and US

Reference

Kinare SG, Parulkar G and Sen PK, Constrictive pericarditis resulting from dracunculosis, Br Med J, March 1962; 1 (5281): 845.

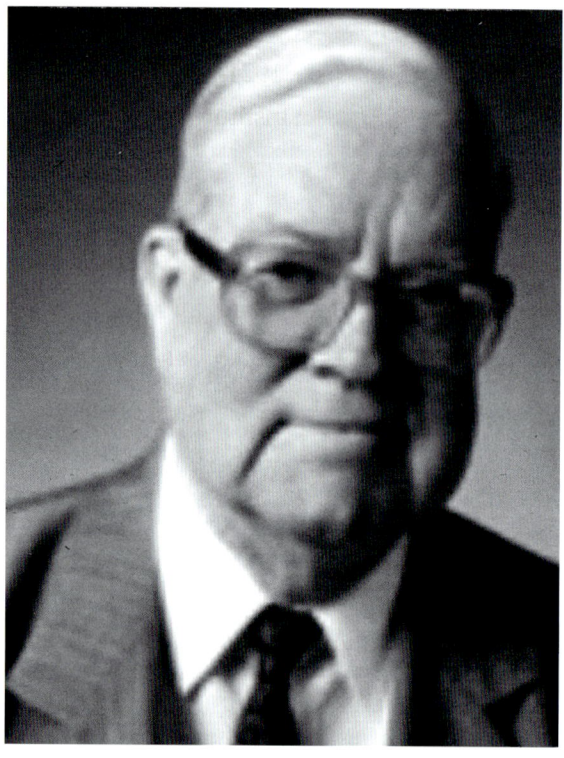

Sven Ivar Seldinger

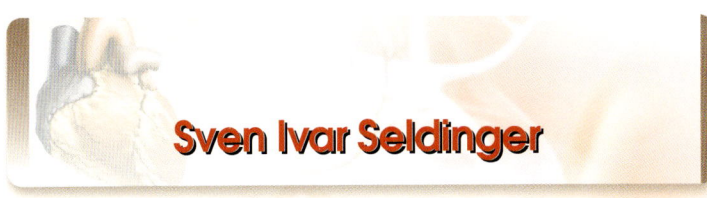

Sven Ivar Seldinger

Dates : 19th April, 1921–1998

Location : Karolinska Institute, Stockholm, Sweden

Contributions

- Introduced the Seldinger technique—percutaneous arterial puncture for angiography
- Performed the first percutaneous renal angiography

Interesting Facts

- First applied a percutaneous technique for cholangiography and for the portal venogaphy
- Received the Valentine award from New York Academy of Medicine

Reference

Seldinger SI, Catheter replacement of the needle in percutaneous arteriography. A new technique, Acta Radiol Suppl (Stockholm), August 2008; 434: 47–52.

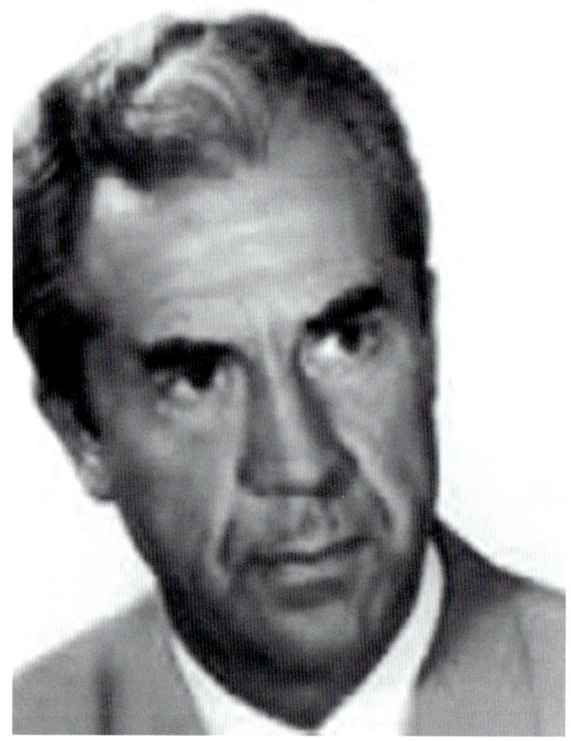

Ake Senning

Reproduced with permission from CTSNet

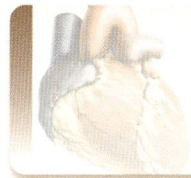

Ake Senning

Dates : 14th December, 1915—21st July, 2000

Location : Karolinska University, Stockholm, Sweden

Chief of Cardiothoracic Surgery, University of Zurich, Switzerland

Contributions

- First open heart surgery with heart lung machine in 1952
- First implantable pacemaker developed with Rune Elmqvist
- Developed fibrillator and defibrillator
- The Senning Operation for TGA—atrial transposition

Interesting Fact

- Trained in orthopedics, trauma and neurosurgery

Reference

Von Segesser LK, Fry M, Senning A, Turina MI, Atrial repair for transposition of the great arteries: Current approach in Zürich based on 24 years of follow-up, Thorac Cardiovasc Surg. Dec. 1991; 39 (Suppl 2): 185–189.

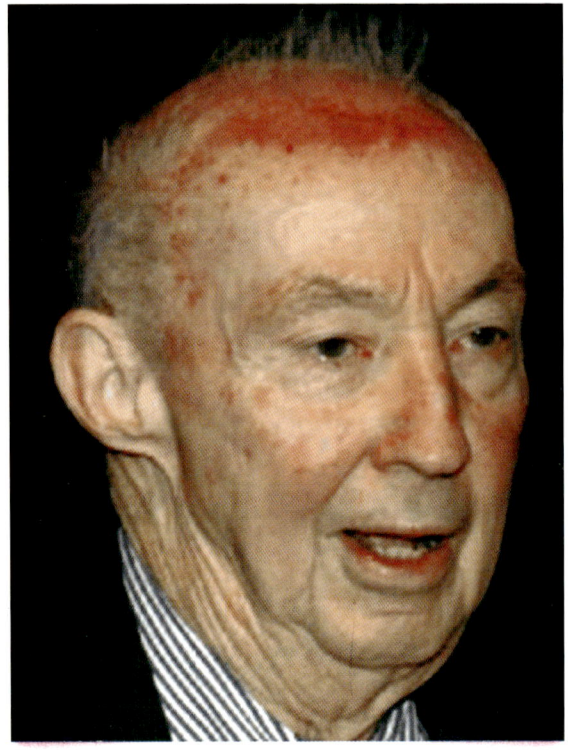

Norman Shumway

Reproduced with permission from CTSNet

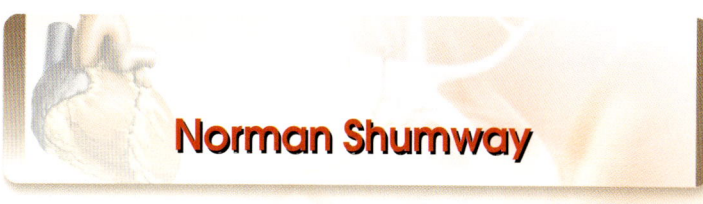

Norman Shumway

Dates : 9th February, 1923–10th February, 2006

Location : Stanford University, San Francisco, USA

Contributions

- The world's second and USA's first successful heart transplant 1968
- The first successful heart lung transplant
- Persevered in developing the program of heart transplantation

Interesting Fact

- Known as one of the Fathers of heart transplantation

Reference

Reitz BA, Burton NA, Jamieson SW, Bieber CP, Pennock JL, Stinson EB, Shumway NE, Heart and lung transplantation: Autotransplantation and allotransplantation in primates with extended survival, J Thorac Cardiovasc Surg 1980; 80: 360–372.

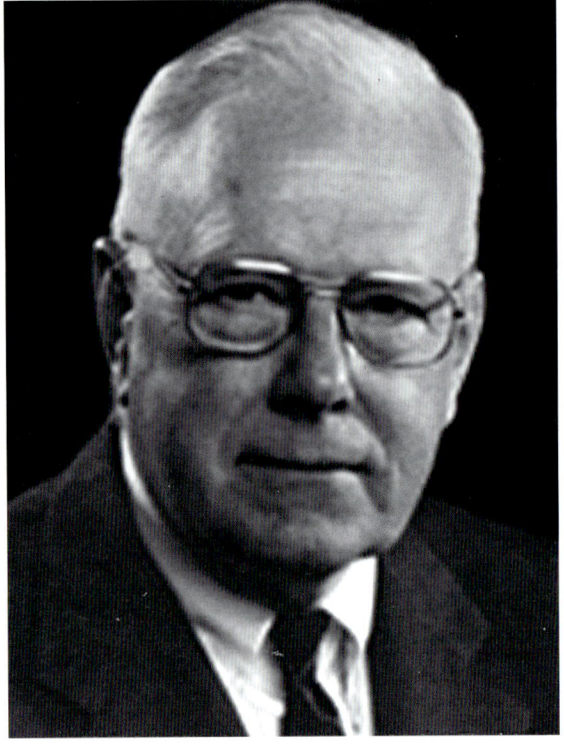

Herbert Sloan

Courtesy of Gerald Rainer

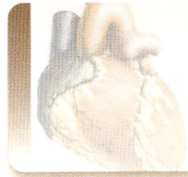

Herbert Sloan

Born : 1914
Location : University of Michigan Medical Centre

Contributions

- The management of thoracic injuries from war wounds.
- Development of thoracic surgical speciality.
- Editor of Annals of Thoracic Surgery.

Interesting Fact

- Avid Gardener with a well nursed flower garden of Rhododendrons.

Reference

Mackenzie JW, Sloan H, MoRms JD, Technic for Correction of Partial Anomalous Pulmonary Venous Insertion and Atrial Septal Defect, Annals of Surg., July 1962; 156(1): 9–11.

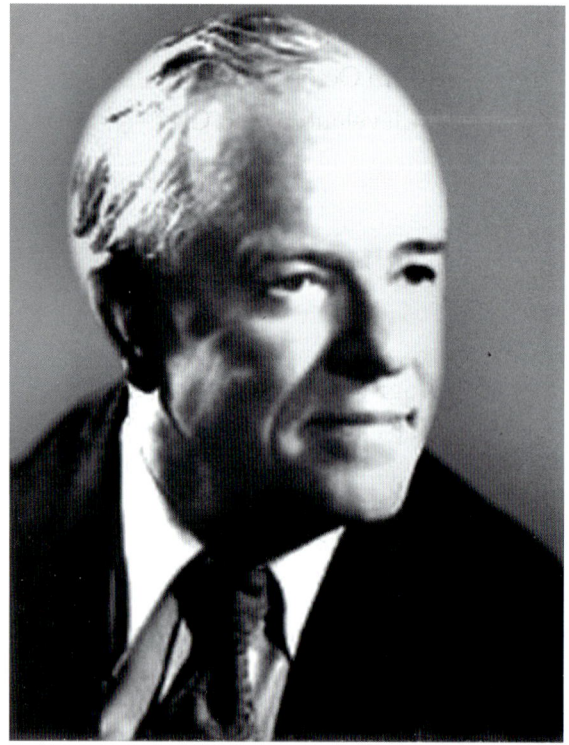

Mason Francis Sones Jr

Reproduced with permission from Wiley Online Library

Mason Francis Sones Jr

Dates : 28th October, 1918 – 28th August, 1985

Location : Cleveland Clinic, Cleveland, Ohio, USA

Contributions

- Introduced for the first time Cardiac Catheterization in neonates in 1954
- Accidentally discovered the technique of selective coronary arteriography in 1958
- Designed cardiac catheter for coronary angiography

Interesting Fact

- Worked with the Kodak Company to develop optical image amplification and designed arteriography equipment.

Reference

Sones FM Jr, Cinecardioangiography, Pediatr Clin North Am, Nov. 1958; 5(4): 945–979.

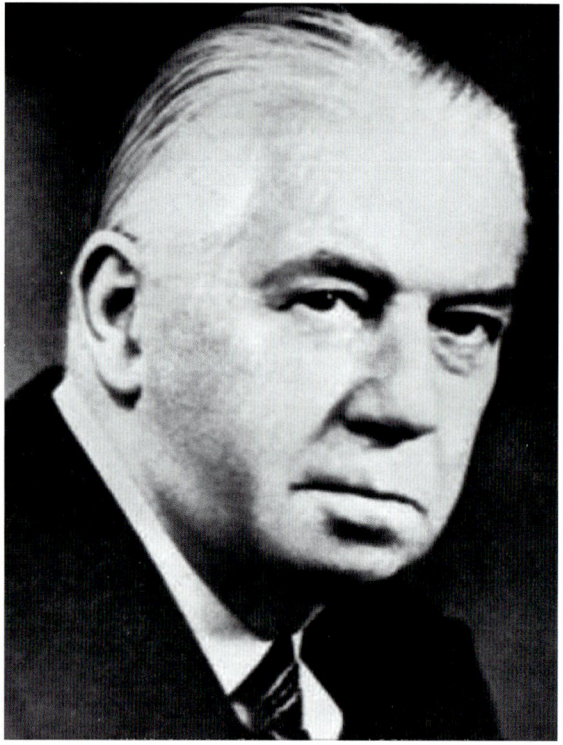

Sir Henry Souttar

Reproduced with permission from Interactive Journal of Cardiovascular Surgery

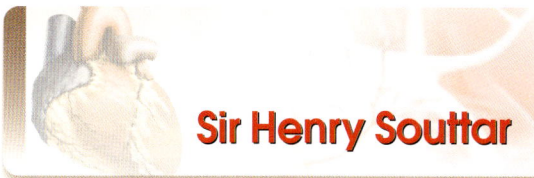

Sir Henry Souttar

Dates : 14th December, 1875–12th November, 1964

Location : The London Hospital, London, UK

Contributions
- In May 1925 he was the first to use a finger to open the mitral valve
- Performed only two such procedures

Interesting Facts
- He was distinguished engineer in India under the British government
- A musician—pianist and violinist

Reference
Souttar HS, The surgical treatment of mitral stenosis, Brit Med J, 1925; 2: 603–606.

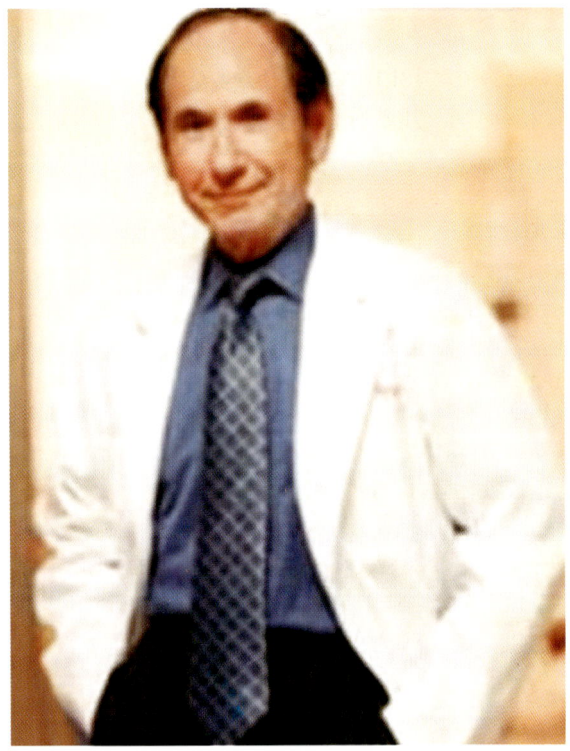

Albert Starr

Indian Journal of Thoracic and Cardiovascular Surgery

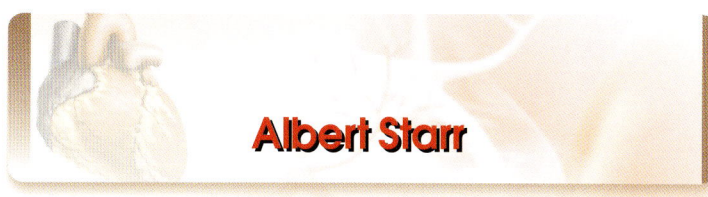

Albert Starr

Born : 1st June, 1926

Location : University of Oregon, Oregon, Washington, USA

Contribution

• Along with Lowell Edwards (Engineer) designed and implanted one of the first artificial valves for replacement of diseased aortic valve in 1961

Interesting Fact

• He moved to Oregon, because he was promised salmon fishing

Reference

Starr A and Edwards ML, Mitral replacement: The shielded ball valve prosthesis, J Thorac Cardiovasc Surg 1961; 42: 673–682.

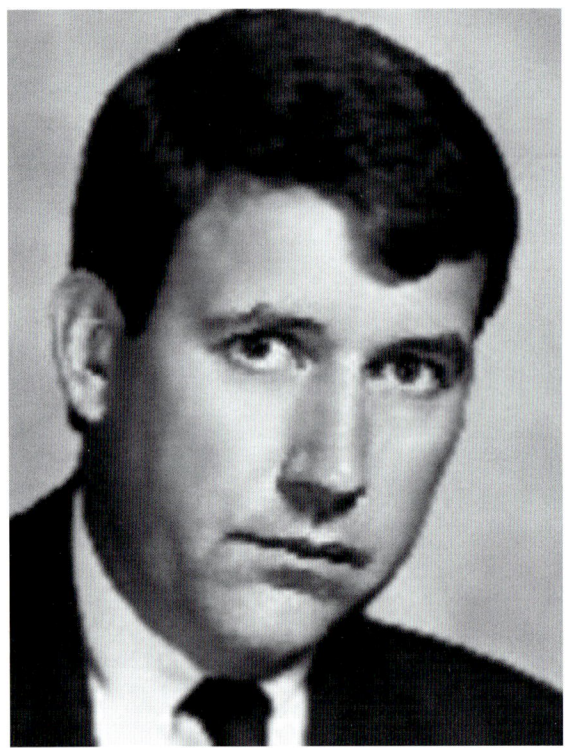

Larry L Stephenson

Reproduced with permission from CTSNet

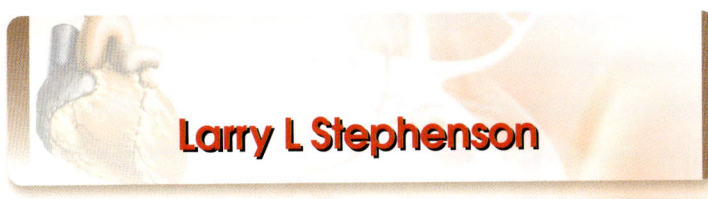

Larry L Stephenson

Born	:	24th February, 1944
Location	:	University of Pennsylvania, Pa
		Wayne State University, School of Medicine, Detroit, Michigan

Contribution

- Described the use of skeletal muscle for cardiac assist

Reference

Patel BG, Shah SH, Astra LI, Hammond RL, Sharif ZA, McDonald PJ, Stephenson LW, Skeletal muscle ventricle aortic counterpulsation: function during chronic heart failure, Ann Thorac Surg, Feb. 2002; 73(2): 588–593.

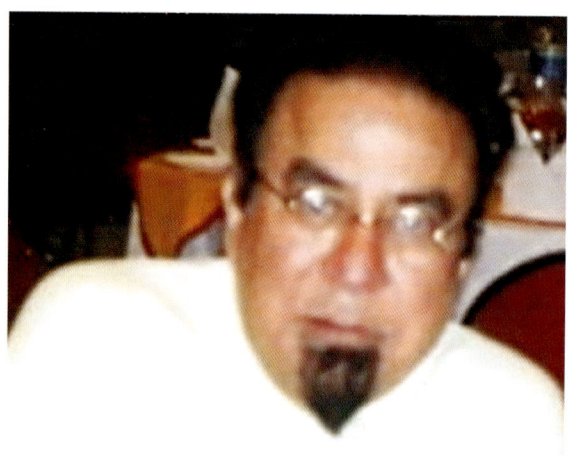

S Subramanian

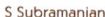

Personal collection

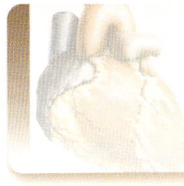

S Subramanian

Born : 8th September, 1933

Location : Buffalo Children's Hospital, Buffalo, NY
Children's Hospital, Tampa, Florida, USA

Contributions

- Total correction of TOF in infancy
- VSD closure under 6 months of age
- Deep hypothermia and circulatory arrest

Interesting Fact

- Born and educated in India

Reference

Subramanian S, Early correction of congenital cardiac defects using profound hypothermia and circulatory arrest, Ann R Coll Surg Engl. April 1974; 54(4): 176–188.

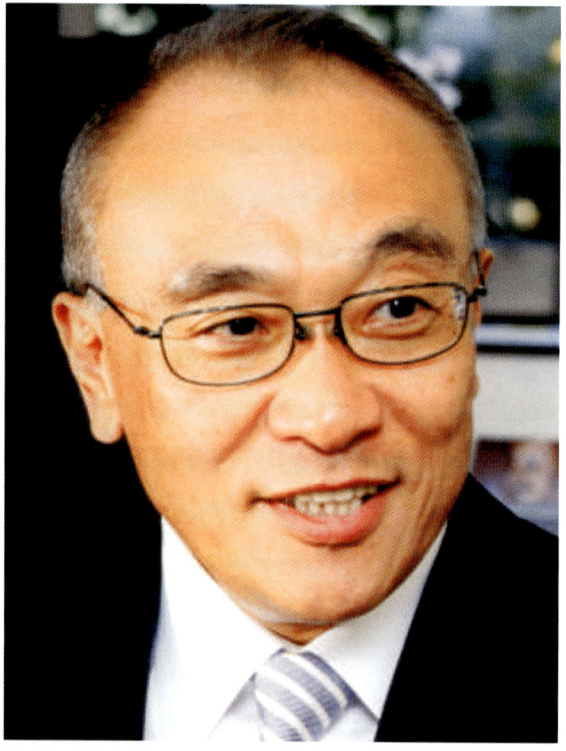

Hisayoshi Suma

Personal collection

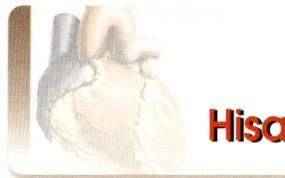

Hisayoshi Suma

Born   :   1st March, 1950
Location   :   The Cardiovascular Institute, Tokyo, Japan

Contribution

- Introduced the technique of using gastroepiploic artery as an arterial conduit for CABG.

Reference

Suma H, Mid-term results for use of the skeletonized gastroepiploic artery graft in coronary artery bypass, Circulation 2007; 71: 1503–1505.

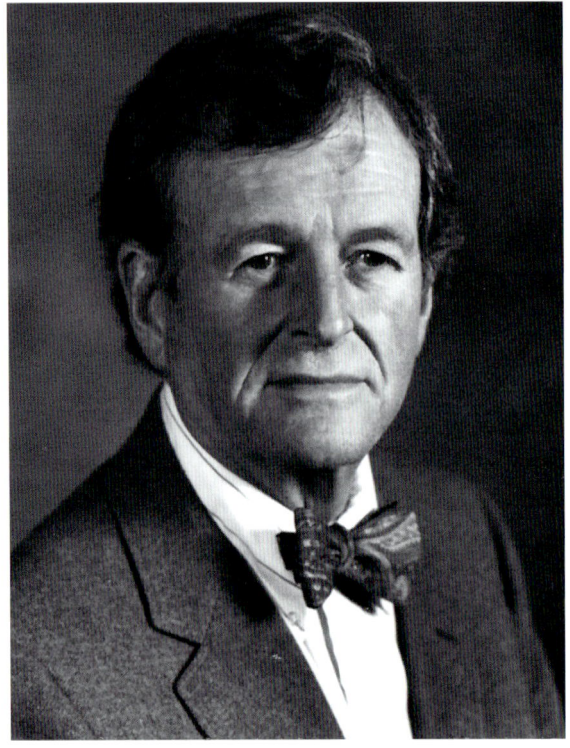

Henry Swan

Courtesy of Gerald Rainer

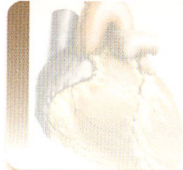

Henry Swan

Born : 1913
Died : July 13, 1996
Location : University of Colorado

Contributions

- Open aortic and pulmonary valvotomy
- The application of hypothermia for cardiac surgery
- Published a large series of open repair of ASD.
- First aortic replacement for aneurysm

Interesting Fact

- Connoisseur of wines, aviator

Reference

Swan H, Virtue RW, Blount SG Jr and Kircher LT Jr, Hypothermia in Surgery: Analysis of 100 Clinical Cases, Ann Surg, September 1955; 142(3): 382–400.

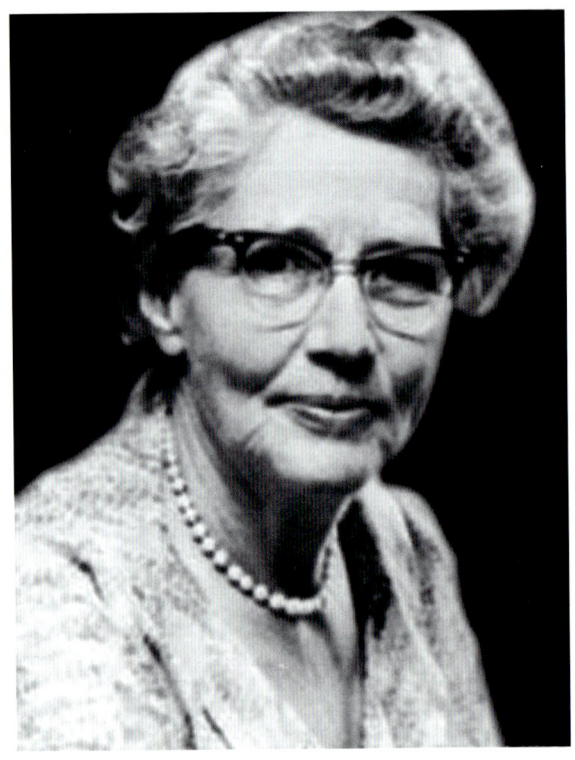

Helen Taussig

Courtesy of Gerald Rainer

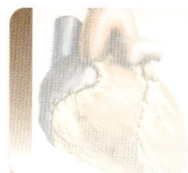

Helen Taussig

Dates	:	24th May, 1898–20th May , 1986
Location	:	Johns Hopkins University, Baltimore, USA

Contributions

- Originator of the idea of a systemic artery pulmonary artery shunt.
- Helped to develop the Blalock Taussig shunt for blue babies, 1944

Interesting Facts

- Was dyslexic
- Helped to stop the use of thalidomide in pregnant women
- President, American Heart Association

Reference

Taussig HB, Talbert J, Bauersfeld R, Swararakrishne, Iyer P, Results of operation for pulmonary stenosis and atresia (Report of 1000 cases), Trans. Ass. Am Phys, 1951; 64: 67–73.

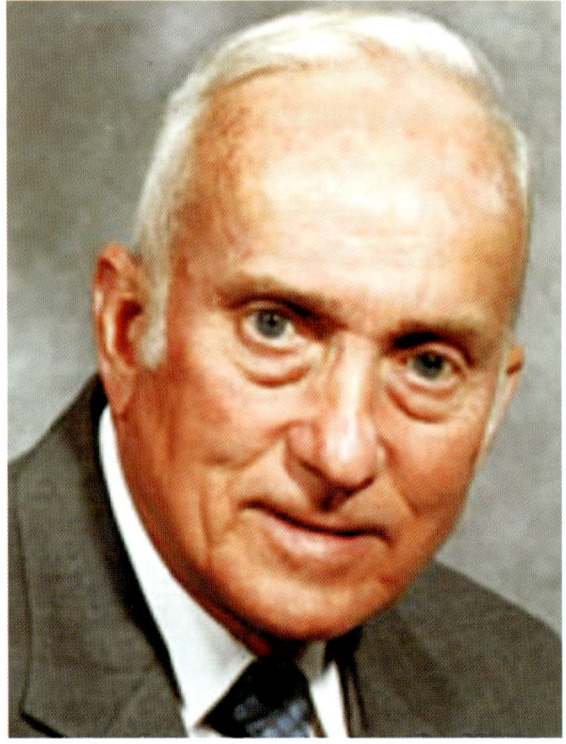

Alfred J Tector

Reproduced with permission from CTSNet

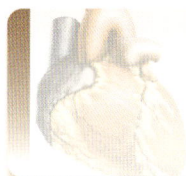

Alfred J Tector

Born : 29th May, 1934

Location : University of Wisconsin, Milwaukee, USA

Cleveland Clinic, Cleveland, Ohio

Contribution

- The technique of sequential grafting with the internal mammary arteries for multiple coronary bypass

Interesting Fact

- Received Wisconsin Historical Society Award May 2008.

Reference

Tector AJ, Decock D, Lepley D, Left main coronary artery occlusion: Surgical management. Cardiovasc Dis. 1974; 1(3): 231–235.

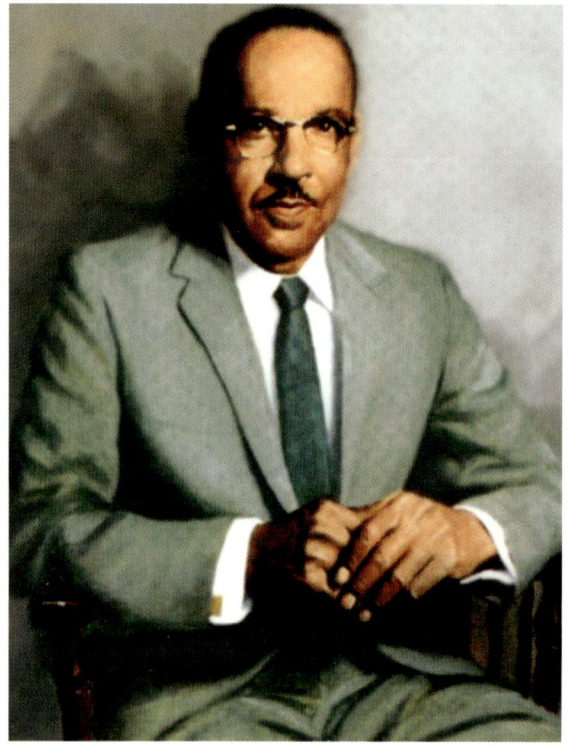

Vivien Theodore Thomas

Courtesy of Dr Duke Cameron, Johns Hopkins Hospital

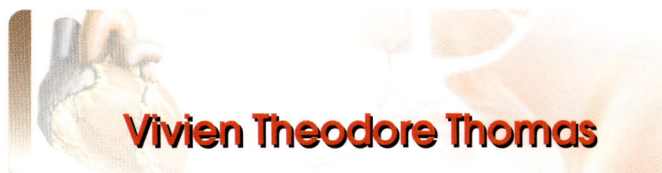

Vivien Theodore Thomas

Dates   : 29th August, 1910–26th November, 1985

Location : Johns Hopkins University, Baltimore, Maryland, USA

Contributions

- A behind the scene pioneer in cardiac surgery who helped Alfred Blalock to perform the Blalock-Taussig shunt, and also the Blalock-Hanlon atrial septectomy for transposition
- Trained a number of cardiac surgeons (including Denton Cooley) in the techniques at Johns Hopkins.

Interesting Facts

- Racial discrimination prevented him from being recognised, during the day he trained surgeons to whom he served drinks in the evening as a Bartender
- He received an honorary Doctorate from Johns Hopkins University

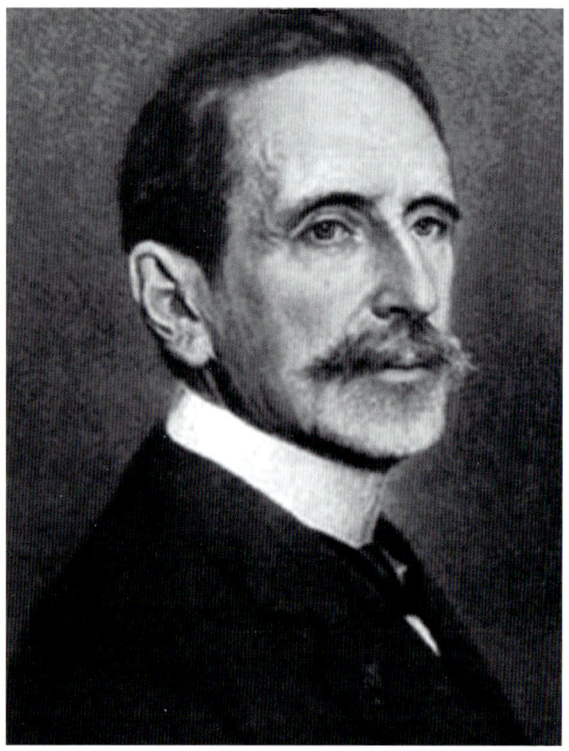

Theodore Tuffier

Reproduced with permission from Interactive Journal of Cardiovascular Surgery

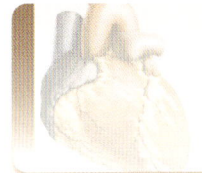

Theodore Tuffier

Dates : 1857–1929

Location : Paris, France

Rockefeller Institute, New York, USA

Contributions

- Tracheal intubation with cuffed tube for ventilation
- The techniques of lung resection
- The method of collapse with plombage

Interesting Facts

- Received surgeon of the highest accomplishment for his efforts during war. Also received Legion of honor and grand cross.

Reference

Tuffier T and Carrel A, Patching and section of the pulmonary orifice of the heart, J Exp Med 1914; 20: 3–8.

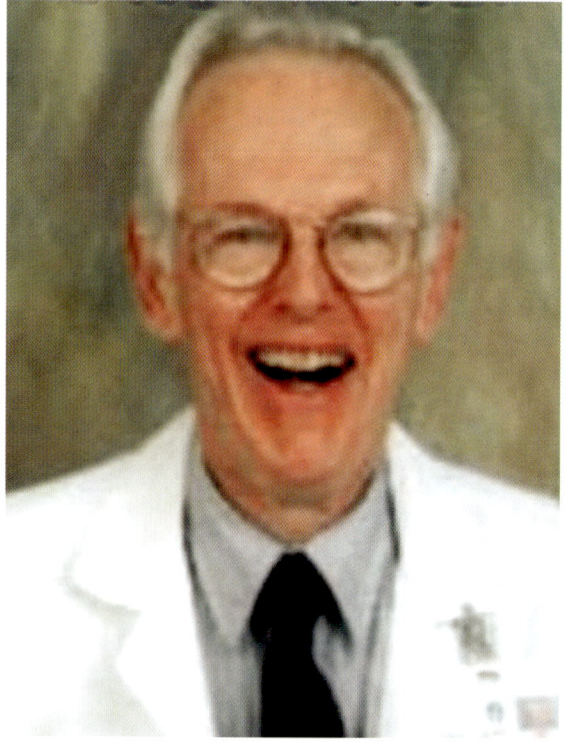

Richard Vanpraagh

Reproduced with permission from Cardiac Registry of Children's Hospital, Boston

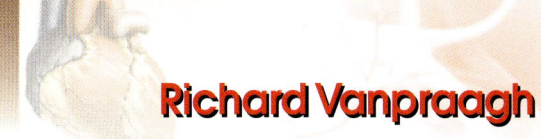

Richard Vanpraagh

Born : 11th April, 1930

Location : Children's Hospital, Harvard University, Boston, Massachusetts, USA

Contributions

- The classical description of many congenital malformations of the heart
- Classification of cardiac anomalies associated with pulmonary stenosis

Interesting Fact

- Together with Stella (his wife), they described new surgical operations

Reference

Praagh RV, Progress in the understanding of congenital heart disease: Double outlet right ventricle (S, D, L) definition of ventriculoarterial discordance, definition of transposition of the great arteries, and the illusion of crisscross AV relations, Texas Heart Inst J, 1988; 15(3): 183–186.

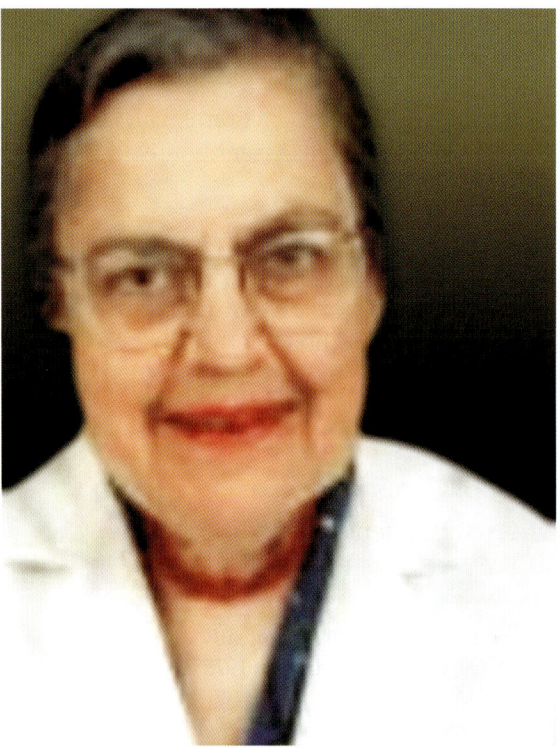

Stella Vanpraagh

Reproduced with permission from Cardiac Registry of Children's Hospital, Boston

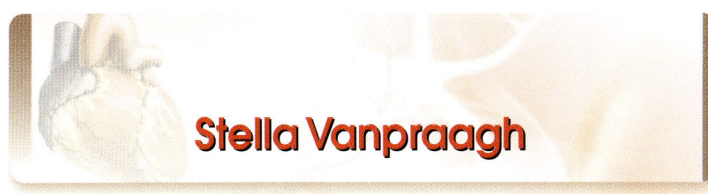

Stella Vanpraagh

Dates : 18th March, 1927–3rd June, 2006

Location : Children's Hospital Medical Centre, Harvard University, Boston, Ma, USA

Contribution

- Pathologist, described and published many interesting congenital malformations of the heart, along with her husband Richard Vanpraagh

Interesting Facts

- Collector of Greek proverbs
- Trained with Helen Taussig

Reference

Praagh RV and Praagh SV, Anatomically corrected transposition of the great arteries, Br Heart J, January 1975; 29(1): 112–119.

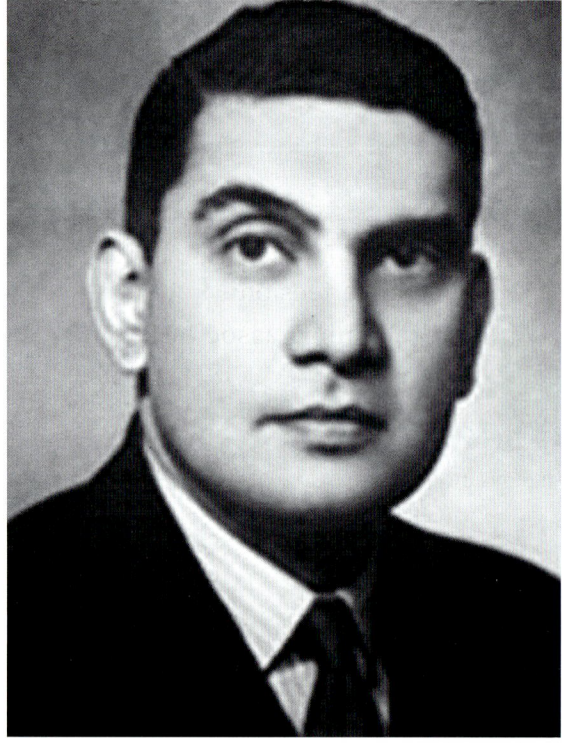

Rustom Jal Vakil

Reproduced with permission from Texas Heart Institute Journal

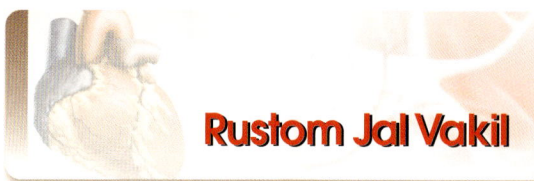

Rustom Jal Vakil

Dates : 17th July, 1911–20th November, 1974

Location : Bombay (Mumbai), India

Contributions

- The introduction of Reserpine (Serpasil) in the management of hypertension
- Recognised syndromes associated with coronary atherosclerosis

Interesting Facts

- Prolific writer, on subjects outside medical practice
- Started a speciality of cardiology in India

Reference

Vakil RJ, A clinical trial of Rauwolfia serpentina in essential hypertension, Br Heart J, October 1949; 11(4): 350–355.

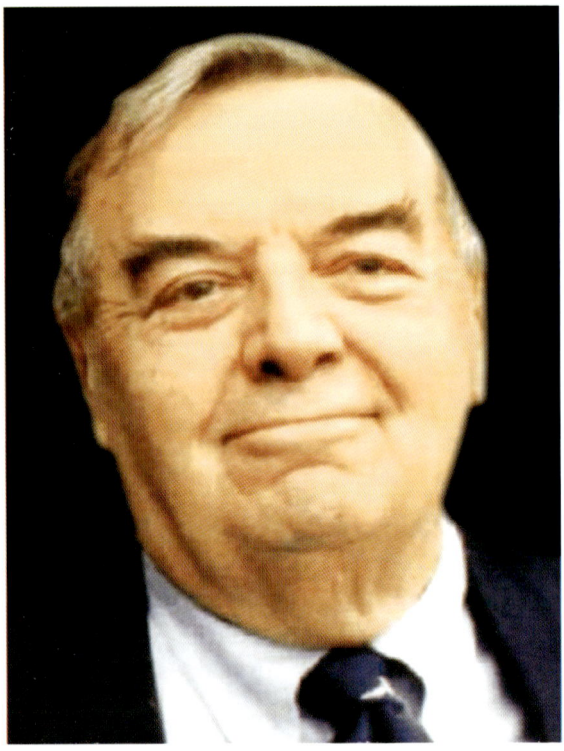

Richard Varco

Reproduced with permission from Annals of Thoracic Surgery

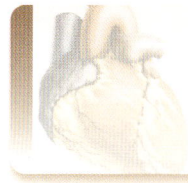

Richard Varco

Dates   : 14th August, 1912–2nd May, 2004
Location : University of Minneapolis, Minnesota, USA

Contributions

- The first successful closure of ASD with John Lewis on September 2, 1952 using the atrial well technique.
- First successful open heart surgery with Walton Lillehei in 1954 with controlled cross circulation
- Coinvented the implantable lung pump
- First successful live donor kidney transplant, development of immunobiology and training two heart transplant pioneers, Norman Shumway and Christian Barnard

Interesting Fact

- "When Dr Varco is done with a case, it looks like the way the Lord made it" a nurse on his team

Reference

Lillehei CW, Cohen M, Warden HE, Read RC, Aust JB, DeWall RA, Varco RL. Direct vision intracardiac surgical correction of tetralogy of Fallot, pentalogy of Fallot and pulmonary atresia defects: Report of first ten cases, Ann. Surg, 1955; 142: 418–442.

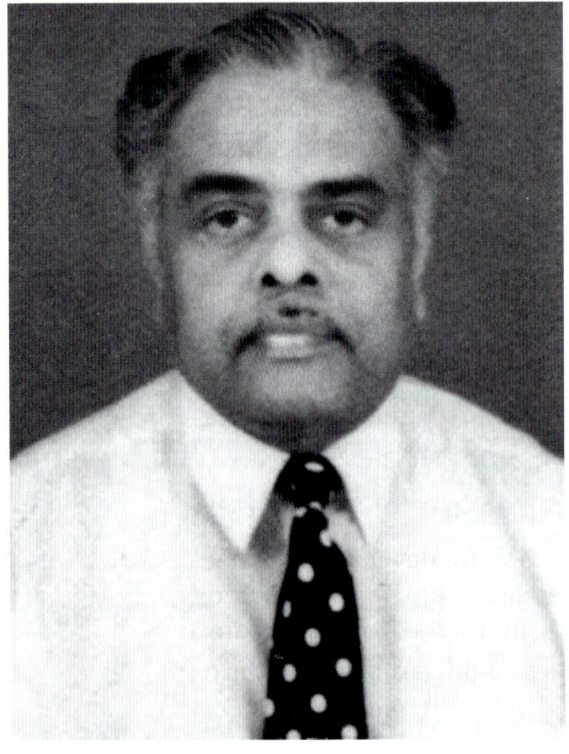

Solomon Victor

Permission from IJTCVS

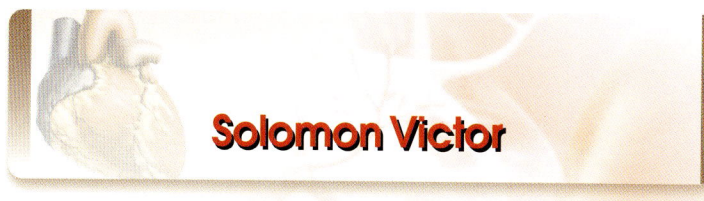

Solomon Victor

Dates : 1938–2006

Location : Madras Medical College and Vijaya Hospital, Chennai, India

Contributions

- The evolution of the human heart and the theory of anticipation
- The anatomy of the mitral and tricuspid valves
- A unique museum of hearts from several marine and mammalian species

Interesting Facts

- Responsible for developing a School Health Programme for detection and prevention of Rheumatic Heart Disease in Chennai and later Tamil Nadu
- He was an avid gardener and the only surgeon with an FRCP

Reference

Victor S and Nayak VM, Evolutionary anticipation of the human heart, Ann R Coll Surg Engl. September 2000; 82(5): 297–302.

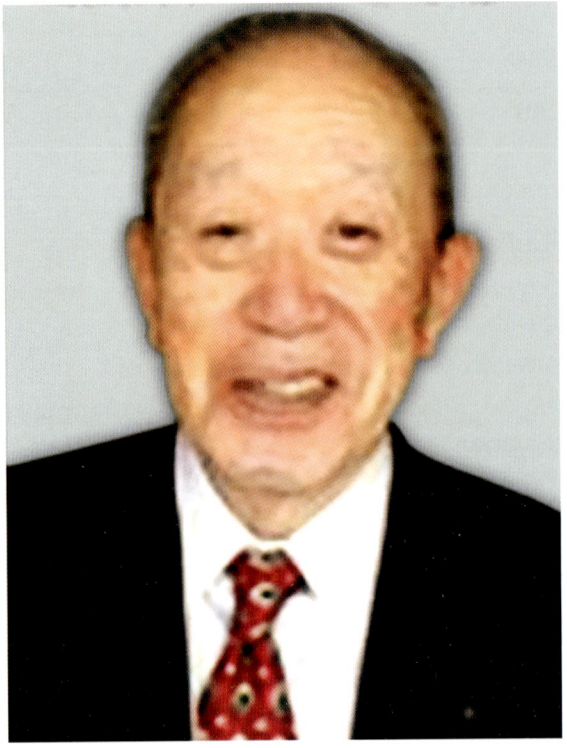

Juro Wada

Reproduced with permission from CTSNet

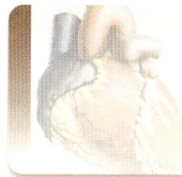

Juro Wada

Dates : 11th March, 1922–14th February, 2011
Location : Sapporo Medical College, Sapporo, Japan

Contribution

- The development of a tilting disc valve. The Wada-Cutter Valve. The second generation valve

Interesting Fact

- Founding member of International Association of Cardiac Surgeons

Reference

Juro W, Sukuzo K, Implantation of heart valve prosthesis and its problems. The Wada hingeless valve, Saishin Igaku 1968; 23: 111–120.

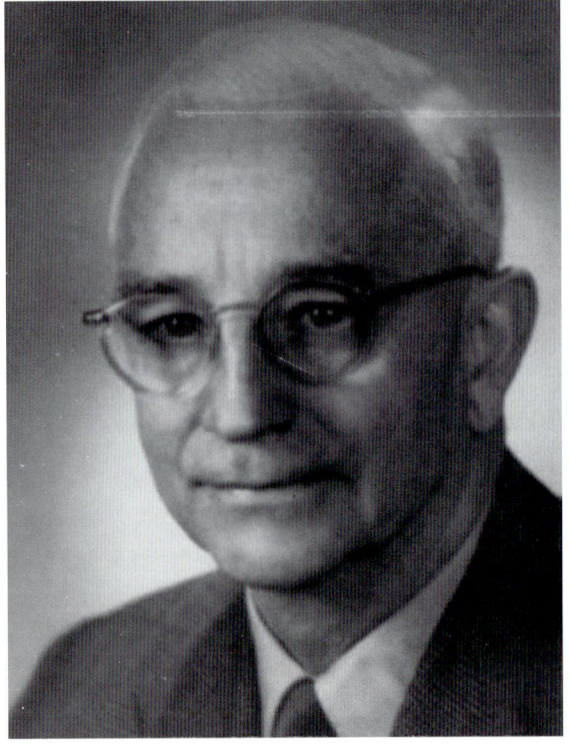

Owen H Wangensteen

Reproduced with permission from Annals of Thoracic Surgery

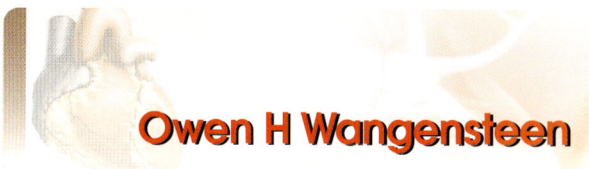

Owen H Wangensteen

Dates   : 1898–1981

Location : University of Minnesota, Minneapolis,
Minnesota, USA

Contributions

- As head of department, spearheaded a program to develop surgical specialities especially open heart surgery and transplantation
- Introduced new suction tube technique for treating intestinal obstruction

Interesting Facts

- It was his vision and encouragement of innovations that led to open heart surgery under direct vision
- Known to have 20 original ideas daily

Reference

Wangensteen OH, Paine JR, Treatment of Acute Intestinal Obstruction by Suction with the duodenal tube, JAMA, 1933; 101 (20): 1532–1539.

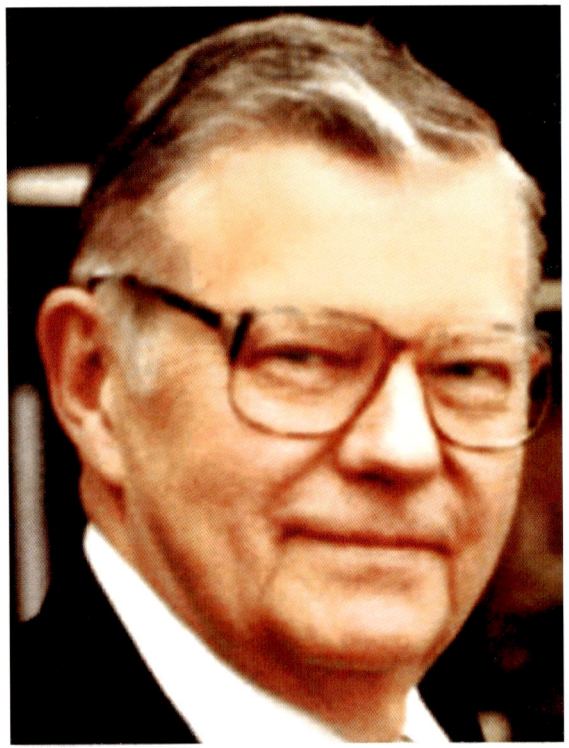

Herbert Edgar Warden

Reproduced with permission from Annals of Thoracic Surgery

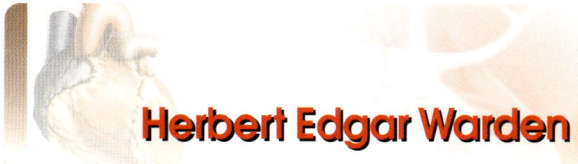

Herbert Edgar Warden

Dates : 30th August, 1920–14th January, 2002
Location : University of Minnesota, Minneapolis
West Virginia University Medical Centre

Contribution

- The first open heart surgery with Walton Lillehei using controlled cross circulation

Interesting Fact

- Was an American football player

Reference

Warden HE, DeWall RA and Varco RL, Use of the right auricle as a pump for the pulmonary circuit, Surg Forum 1954; 5: 16–22.

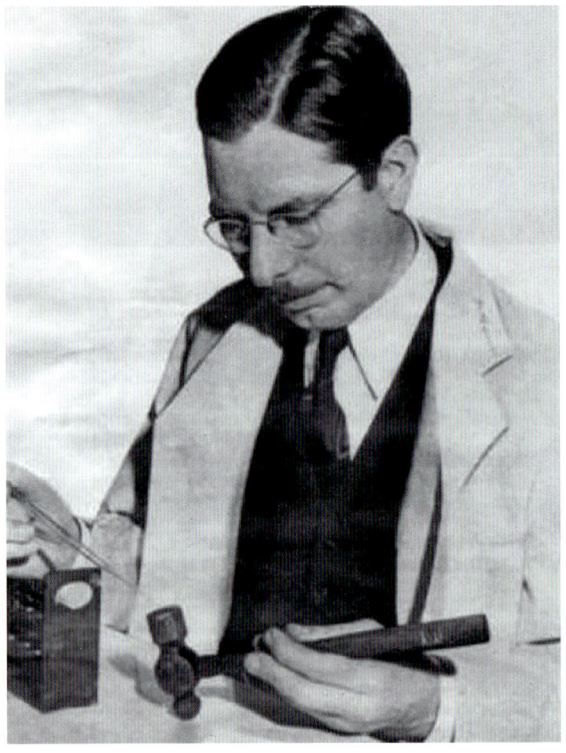

Alexander Weiner

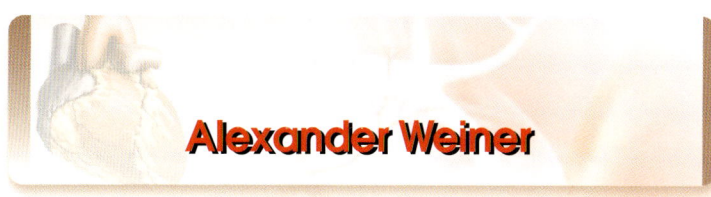

Alexander Weiner

Dates : 1907–1976
Locations : New York, USA

Contribution

- Along with Karl Landsteiner in 1957 discovered the blood groups and Rh factor which revolutionised blood transfusion

Interesting Fact

- Received the Lasker Award in 1946 for this pioneering work

Reference

Landsteiner K and Weiner AS, Studies on an agglutinogen (Rh) in human blood reacting with anti-rhesus sera and with human isoantibodies, J Exp Med, September 1941; 74(4): 309–320.

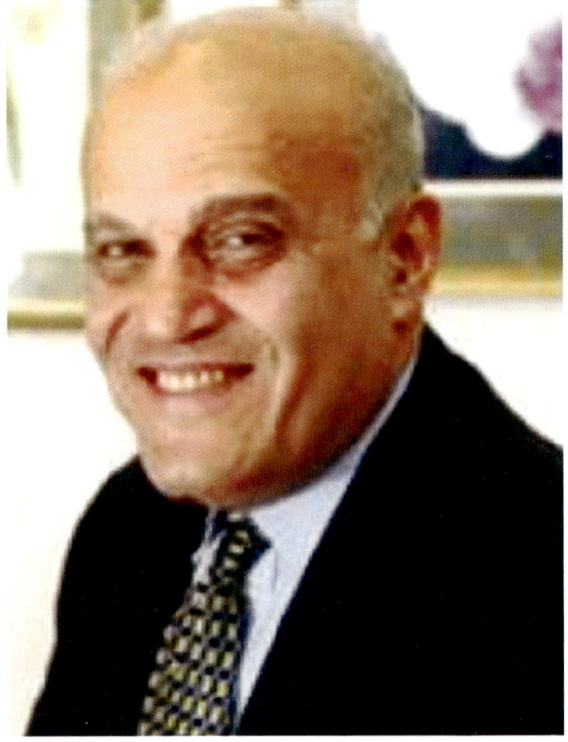

Sir Magdi Habib Yacoub

Personal collection

Sir Magdi Habib Yacoub

Born : 1935

Location : Harefield Hospital and Imperial College, London, UK

Contributions

- First heart lung transplants in the world
- Most experienced transplant surgeon in the UK
- First pediatric heart transplant

Interesting Facts

- Knighted by the queen in 1991
- Philanthropist—started the Chain of Hope charity

Reference

Yacoub MH, Smith RR and Hilton CJ, Anatomical correction of complete transposition of the great arteries and ventricular septal defect in infancy, Brit Med J. 1976; 1: 1111–1116.

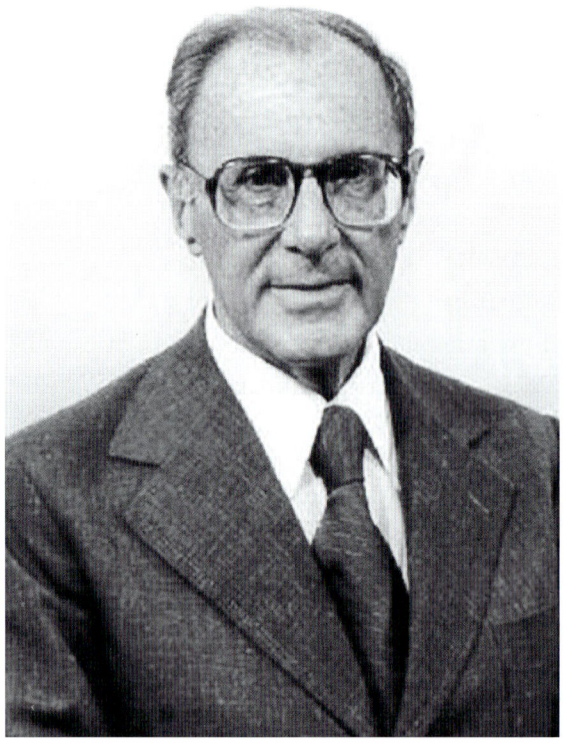

Euriclydes de Jesus Zerbini

Euriclydes de Jesus Zerbini

Dates : 17th May, 1912–23rd October, 1993

Location : Sao Paulo, Brazil

Contributions

• Pioneered the heart surgery program, closed and open heart in Brazil

• Developed a ball and cage valve with Adib Jatene

• Introduced the dura mater valves—tissue valve preserved in glycerol

Interesting Fact

• His Motto "Hard Work Never Hurt"

Reference

Puig LB, Verginelli G, Belotti G, Kawabe L, Frack CC, Pileggi F, Décourt LV, Zerbini EJ, Homologous dura mater cardiac valve. Preliminary study of 30 cases, J Thorac Cardiovasc Surg. July 1972; 64(1): 154–160.

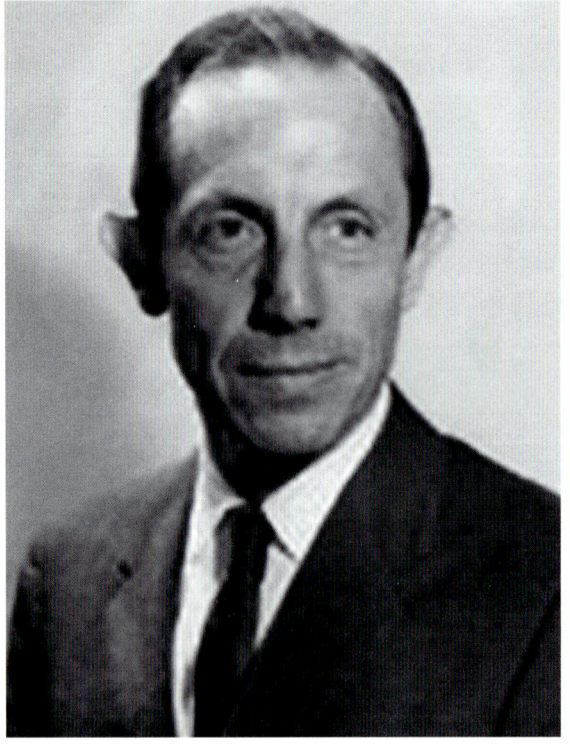

Paul Maurice Zoll

Internet/Wikipedia

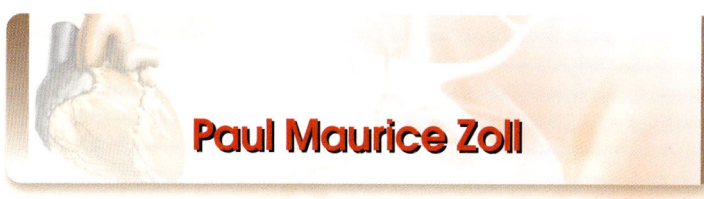

Paul Maurice Zoll

Dates : 15th July, 1911–8th January, 1999

Location : Beth Israel Hospital, Harvard University, Boston, Massachusetts, USA

Contributions

- The pioneer who invented the pacemaker, a large device that could help the heart by stimulation
- Developed the defibrillator

Interesting Fact

- His work and his inventions were considered unethical and dangerous

Reference

Zoll PM, Resuscitation of the heart in ventricular standstill by external electrical stimulation, NEJM, 1952; 247: 768–771.

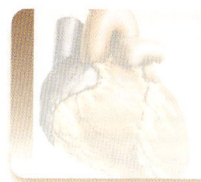

Index